iii

# Table of Contents

How You Manage Your Money
Evaluating the Dynamics of Your Marital/Family Atmosphere

# Introduction

*Why This Book and Why Now?*

Obesity in America has soared in the past few decades in spite of advancement in bariatric technology, information on nutrition, fancy exercise equipment, or more efficient exercise routine used to keep your body in motion.  As I received instructions from God concerning this book, it didn't take me long to realize it is designed to get the body of Christ off the world system when it comes to your health.  The principles within this book are aligned with kingdom principles that results in divine health.  Here's the good news for non-believers, you will reap the same results when you apply these principles in your own life.  In addition to this good news, it's not too late to accept His gift of salvation (Jesus Christ) and avoid spending eternity in Hell.

Witnessing the escalation of these perilous times reveals the brokenness of our world systems. The judicial system is broken, the financial system is broken, and the healthcare system is most definitely broken. Now is your window of opportunity to establish your independence from all the world systems.  My assignment within the body of Christ is to help His people disconnect from the healthcare system.  Transcending to divine health will establish your independence from:  medications, lifestyle induced surgeries, organ transplants and artificial body parts & organs.  You see my friend; this level of health is possible in the Kingdom of God.

*Using My Life as Your Learning Curve*

I now realize how God methodically used all my past experiences (good & bad) and weight loss challenges to prepare me for such a time as these.  As I've matured in my walk with Him, He revealed to my spirit many secrets hidden "for" us and not "from" us as believers. I eventually came to realize a deeper understanding of the model prayer Jesus taught the disciples in Matthew 6: 10 as it reads, "...your kingdom come, your will be done, on earth as it is in heaven." God desires the earth to operate just like things operate in heaven.  In heaven, there is no poverty, no fear, no darkness, no sickness and most definitely no obesity.  In other words, earth is supposed to mirror

Published in the United States by Amazon.com
www.Amazon.com

Trina Claiborne
The Kingdom of God Permanent Weight Loss Principles
Biblical references are New International Version (NIV)
ISBN 978-0-9988210-3-0
eISBN 978-0-9988210-1-6
Audio ISBN 978-0-9988210-6-1
Printed in the United States of America
Designed by Trina Claiborne

**Also by Trina Claiborne**
**How I Lost 40 Pounds in 90 Days While Traveling**
**Operation:  Life Re-Map for Divine Health Workbook**
*(The companion to The Kingdom of God Permanent Weight Loss Principles)*

## * * Dedication * *

As an ambassador of the Kingdom of God, I dedicate this book on behalf of the King to the Body of Christ *(BOC)* first, and to whosoever willing to hear and accept His words of truth. The manifestation of this book is the fruit of my faith in God's mandate I received to deliver His blueprint on how to walk in divine health. His desire is to return our faith back to His government where anything and everything is possible for those that believe in Him.

Because our society has made major advancement in technology and increased in knowledge; we are living longer but with major health complications being sustained predominantly by medication, artificial limbs and organs. God wants you to know He has a better plan, and the side effect is a life of divine health.

We are living in perilous times, but compared to what's about to come upon the earth; the Body of Christ, and anyone that has an ear to hear; must live a life independent of the world's health system to withstand the coming storms.

As an author and healthy lifestyle coach, I pledge never to present a healthy lifestyle problem without presenting a Kingdom solution.


In Good Health,

Trina Claiborne, Author & Healthy Lifestyle Coach

heaven.  My weight loss journey and matured personal relationship with Jesus Christ revealed to me that being overweight has spiritual factors as the root cause.  Many non-believers fail to realize human beings are a spirit, living temporary in an earth suit called "a body". Your body is made of three parts:  Mind, Body and Soul; which have the power to physically manifest the condition of your spirit.  God as your creator gave you His spirit and your spirit is always searching for spiritual food through and from His word.  When you feed your spirit anything inconsistent with the word of God, it begins to reflect in your body as failing health and for many; excessive body fat.  God gave you His word in the **B**asic **I**nstructions **B**efore **L**eaving **E**arth testament (aka the "BIBLE), and sent the Holy Spirit to dwell within you as a guide and a comforter sent straight from heaven.   This revelation led me to examine common weight loss principles to discover the comparison to Kingdom principles for divine health. Understanding everything on earth has principles automatically include principles for permanent weight loss.  In addition to revealing kingdom weight loss principles, this book also reveal the elements required to help you construct "how" to implement these principles into your life; regardless of your life's complexities.

This book is the guide to help you complete the workbook entitled "Operation:  Life Re-Map for Divine Health; as you discover the external factors contributing to your current state of being. Beloveth, you have the power to voluntarily remove these factors through a gift from God called "Freedom of Choice".   This gift can be your best friend or your worst enemy, and the good news is you get to choose your path.  Your mind is a very powerful, complex system designed to provoke action based on your beliefs.   This book is designed to transform your belief to line up with God's promises for your life.  For this reason, the solutions to your weight loss journey starts with revealing a picture of your truth.  The next phase starts with your spirit flowing outward to external factors and eventually ending full circle with a new commitment from your spirit.

My life experiences and weight loss journey established two truths that set me free:

1. **Everything that exists in the natural was first created in and by the spirit.**
2. **The human body is extremely complex, but 100% predictable when it comes to weight loss.**

My desire is for you to embrace these truths to set you free from your weight loss challenges and "all" the contributing factors that kept you losing your weight loss battle over the years.

# Part I – Enlightenment of Truths

## Chapter 1: *The Truth about Obesity*

Brace yourself because this may be very difficult for many of you. Grab a mirror or get in front of a mirror and chant this phrase out loud: I *(state your name)* am responsible for my reflection in the mirror! Again, I *(state your name)* am responsible for my reflection in the mirror! One more time! I *(state your name)* am responsible for my reflection in the mirror! I realize chanting that phrase out loud three times make your skin crawl, and possibly saying to yourself "how dare Trina think I'm responsible for looking the way I look and feeling the way I feel! Well guess what? I did because it's true. Here's the good news; because you are responsible, you're also the solution and has the power to change it. I do understand your frustration because I felt the same way when this revelation was revealed to me a few years back about myself. So don't throw this book across the room just yet. This next statement is the truth for every living person on the planet. Every single thing you do from the moment you get up until you lay your head down to sleep is either getting you closer to ultimate health or taking you farther from it. You are making that choice every single day conscientiously or unconscientiously, and either method has a predictable outcome.

Let's start this journey with understanding what obesity is. According to the American Heart Association, obesity applies to individuals who are more than 20% above the normal body weight. During my research on obesity these two words appeared quite a bit, "epidemic' and "disease". So I wanted to know the true meaning of these two words in order to get a better understanding of what the industry 'experts' are saying about obesity that's shaping your mindset concerning obesity. The word epidemic according to Webster's dictionary is defined as; affecting or tending to affect a disproportionately large number of individuals within a population, community or region at the same time. The word disease is defined as a disorder or incorrectly functioning organ, part, structure or system of the body resulting from the effect of genetic or development errors.

These conditions can lead to: infection, nutritional deficiency or imbalances, illness, sickness, or ailment. Webster also included unfavorable environmental factors that can lead to toxicity or poison that will cause a disease. So according to this definition in order to be deemed a disease there has to be a disorder or malfunction of the body. I wanted to know the true meaning of these words simply because I've been reading time and time again that obesity is a disease and it has become an epidemic. Gathering this information led me to get a better understanding of a few more words like: habits and addictions.

Before I dive into the definition of habits, I want to share some information that was revealed to me from my spiritual father Myles Munroe a Pastor out of the Bahamas; may he now rest in peace. In one of his teachings, he revealed the importance of time. He states, "Time is a commodity used to buy life, and what you do with your time becomes your life!" Now that's some wisdom no man on the planet can deny. Now that we have a clear understanding about the importance of time, let's look at habits. A habit is referred to routine behavior that is repeated regularly and has the tendency to occur consciously or subconsciously. There are two important things you must understand about habits. Habits have the ability to eat up time and always produce an expected end. For example, if you smoke regularly for the past 10-20 years and get diagnosed with lung cancer; you should not be a shock. If you constantly hang out with friends at a bar drinking and having a good time four to five times a week over a five year period; don't expect to become the owner of an international billion dollar company. Why; because those habits does not lead to that, but you can expect to develop into an alcoholic. So beloved, if you decide to increase your daily water intake, exercise more regularly, eat less calories than you burn off and eat more fresh or fresh frozen foods; you will experience better health and weight loss. You see a habit can be your worst enemy or your best friend. If you can figure out the results you want operating in your life, then let that knowledge dictates your habits.

Now let's get a better understanding of addictions. According to Psychology Today, an addiction is a condition that results when a person ingests a substance regularly or engages in a pleasurable activity where continued use can becomes compulsive and interferes with ordinary life responsibilities such as; work, relationships and health.

Now that we have a better understanding of obesity, epidemics, disease, habits and addictions we can now pull it all together to see what they reveal about the truth. The true revelation is obesity has become an epidemic because too many of us have adapted the same lifestyle, and it leads to the same result; obesity. Food is a wonderfully dangerous thing. It keeps us alive and it also has the ability to lead to death and disease when abused. Food addiction is the worst addiction to have because you can't live without it. What I'm about to say concerning addiction is not likely embraced by religious people *(none-Kingdom mind-set)* or non-believers of the Faith. I truly believe addictions are man's attempt to fill a spiritual void with a tangible substance. Here's the problem; because these types of voids are spiritual, they can only be satisfied with spiritual things, and using anything else just won't do! That's why an addict escalates in abusing the drug of their choice. As you already know food is not the only vice people use in attempt to fill spiritual voids. Many chose illegal drugs, alcohol, sex, smoking, shopping, or working too much; which will bring temporary pleasure, but over time they become numb to it and need more to attain or maintain that level of pleasure. That's why food is the most dangerous addiction to have because you can't live without it. The biggest challenge a food addict must overcome is learning to relate to food differently. I don't have any facts to back up this next statement, but it's my personal belief based on wisdom and understanding, many food addicts choose food as their drug of choice simply because it's portable; you can't get arrested for having it in your possession; it will not impair driving; unless you're driving in Atlanta, GA traffic; you can purchase it anywhere and lastly it taste so good!

Adapting daily habits of eating more calories than you burn off has an expected end of weight gain; this process is clearly not a malfunction. Your body is simply responding to the demands you're placing upon it; therefore, obesity is not a disease. I realize it may feel that I went around to mountain to come to this point, but it is very important that you understand obesity is not disease. Believing obesity is a disease takes away your accountability of being responsible for your weight. If obesity is a disease; that means a 115 pound person could wake up one morning and weight 215 pounds overnight: Why? Because they contracted obesity. Now that's meshuga; pronounced "Ma-Sugah", a Jewish word for crazy.

# Chapter 2: *The True Dynamics of a Creator*

I want to warn you, if you believe the existence of mankind is the result of evolution or the big bang theory; you're not going to feel warm and fuzzy about this chapter. If you are brave enough, give me a minute to explain. Let's begin by understanding the mind of a creator; independent of religious beliefs. Why does a creator create anything? I think that's a great question because in today's world, things are changing so rapidly it's hard to keep up. You can purchase a computer today, and in three months or less it's obsolete. Why; because the next "creator" has figured out a way to make it better. Creators create for two dominant reasons: 1. to solve an existing problem with a new product or service to get better results or improve the process. 2: to improve the function of a process or equipment already in existence. You may be the creator of a product or service or know someone that is, and all creators have this in common: they never create anything without the ability built within the thing to perform what it was created for. I hope you heard what I just said! A creator NEVER creates anything without putting the ability in the thing, to perform the purpose for which it was created for. Here is where I want to give a word of knowledge and wisdom to evolutionist. When you look at the species called "man", it is a very complex creature and designed with extreme structure & very organized. No one on the planet can go inside a lab and create a man from scratch. I'm not talking about harvesting an egg from a woman or a sperm from a man then putting it in a peach dish. I'm talking about creating man out of nothing existing in the natural realm. When you look at mankind closely, you can clearly see that every body part has a purpose. For instance, your eyes were conveniently placed on the front of your head close to the brain giving you the ability to see not only where you go, but to avoid obstacles. Imagine if your eyes were placed on the bottom of your foot. Even your nose hair has a purpose; it blocks or traps debris from entering your nasal passage while breathing. Now if each body part has a purpose, we can surely deduct the whole person has a purpose for living. So I now ask you, what are the chances of man coming into existence due to some random transformation or some explosion causing elements to come together to create a man with this level of precision and organization? If you believe that's possible, then you also can believe a coke bottle came into existence by the random formation of glass that exploded into the shape of a coke bottle; and red & white paint somehow found its way to the bottle and form the words "Coca Cola", and the bottles somehow made its way into the homes of people and businesses all over the world.  You are talking about an*other meshuga moment!* I want to share this to assure we are on the same page; understanding that mankind not only had to be created, but have a purpose based on those simple wisdom keys.  So let's get started and discover your purpose!  .

# Part II
## The Kingdom of God Permanent Weight Loss Principles

### Chapter 3:  Two Foundational Truths for Permanent Weight Loss

The events that led me to these foundational truths started when I read the bible and received a deeper spiritual understanding of God as our creator.  If you've read the bible with spiritual understanding, God's desire for your life is not a mystery.  John the apostle was the author of John from the four gospels, 1st, 2nd & 3rd John and Revelations.  In 3rd John 1: 2, he writes, "Dear friend, I pray that you may enjoy good health and that all may go well with you, even as your soul is getting along well."  As a believer of "The Faith", I've read this passage many times just like many other believers.  Without spiritual understanding, it appears to be a simple letter John writes to his friend Gaius.  In reality, he was operating as a messenger of God, decreeing God's desire for them to not only walk in divine health, but to prosper in every area of their life including their soul.  Although non-believers in the faith may not know, most of the New Testament comprised of letters written to the churches by an ex-Christian serial killer named Saul; who was renamed Paul by Jesus Christ on the road to Damascus.  As a believer in the "faith", you are the church; therefore, these letters apply directly to you personally.  It is my desire to share what God revealed to my spirit; as we mature in our walk with Him, we develop a deeper relationship that reveals a deeper understanding of His words, easier access to His promises, a clearer picture of His character and a deeper understanding of Him as "The Great I AM".  You see my friend, the word of God is extremely pregnant and when He said in Hosea 4: 6, "...My people are destroyed from a lack of knowledge." I've come to know that statement is loaded.  When God created the earth and mankind out of His spirit as the spoken word, His desire was to create a family that operates on earth just as things operate in heaven.  In heaven, everything is operated and controlled by love and full of life; remember there are no sickness, no death, no darkness, no poverty, no stress, and no fear in heaven.  Here's the lesson in all of this, God is a spirit and His words are spirit.  He made us in His image; therefore, we are spirits, our words are spirits, and spirits create that which is spoken. I felt compelled to rewrite that statement to resonate within you. God made you in His image; therefore, you are a spirit, your words are spirits, and spirits create that which is spoken. How can we know that? I think that's a great question! If you haven't already, grab your bible and take a look at Genesis 1 starting with the later part of verse two. As the Spirit of God was hovering over the waters, He started speaking and commanding from verse 2 through verse 30, and finally in verse 31; He saw all that He spoke in a manifested form, and it was very good. See the pattern? God's words manifested that which was spoken in the natural realm. Now, take a moment to exam your life, and the fruits produced by your words. Your words give shape to how you spend your time, the quality of your thoughts and the actions you take as a result. I encourage you to examine how your words have produced your current experiences in your weight loss journey, your health, your finance, your family, your friends, your ministry, your job or business. I pray you seriously take this time to be totally honest with yourself because in order to help yourself, you must be honest with yourself. I realize this examination may be a little difficult because sometimes the external voices in your life can be so loud it's hard to hear or pay attention to what you've been repeating in your own head or notice what's been coming out of your mouth.

Here's another faucet of creation most believers and definitely non-believers miss. When God spoke mankind into existence, *(Genesis 1: 26)* he gave ruler-ship over the earth to man and not to Himself. WOW, what a bold move! From a "natural" understanding, it appears that God just created Himself a massive problem; ...but did He? The answer to that is No, and absolutely not! When God said, "Let us make man in our own image and our likeness", it's important to discover what is the image and likeness of God? As we noted earlier, God is a spirit and not a human as stated in Numbers 23: 19. God is love *(1ˢᵗ John 4: 8),* and that means mankind is a spirit walking around in an earth suit that's designed for love, to be loved and to give love. This spirit God placed inside of you is His supernatural way of communicating with you from heaven. As a matter of fact, we *(mankind)* are the only created being God gave a spirit and we are the only created being He gave dominion over the earth.  Just because Satan was slick enough to steal it from us temporarily, did not negate God's desire to get that authority back into the hands of mankind. Because God is love and He love us so much, He became a man through the birth of Jesus carrying His spirit *(aka "The Christ")* to make Himself legal to operate on earth as a man.  Jesus' shed blood purchased back "EVERYTHING" Satan stole from mankind, and that my dear is loaded with so many benefits that it requires a mature spirit to understand it all.

As a healthy lifestyle coach, I wanted to share this spiritual understanding to help you see who you truly are, the authority you have, how it relates to what you see in the mirror, and how you feel emotionally & spiritually.  Remember earlier I stated my coaching sessions are based on this 1st statement of truth:  **"Everything that exists in the natural was first created in and by the spirit."** As I conduct my coaching sessions upon this truth, it's important to help you understand just how dominating your spirit is over every area of your life.  In addition to being a spirit, you possess a soul that's comprised of your mind; your *thought life.*  I believe as you read this book or listen to the audio you'll begin to understand your mind and thoughts are shaped by what you see and what you hear.  Your eyes and ears are the gateway to your mind and soul.  That's how faith comes and that's how faith grows, by hearing the word of God as it settles in your heart. Faith is the ability to "**see**" the promises in the spiritual realm **and speak it** "BEFORE" it's manifested in the natural realm.  Once you see or hear a thing, it's the belief or meaning you give to create an emotion; and that emotion will dictate your action(s). When you walk by sight, your actions will be based on what you physically see, but when you walk by faith; your action will be based on the truth God said in His word regardless of what you see.  This kingdom principle is reflected in two verses: Romans 10: 17 – "Consequently, **faith comes** from hearing the message, and the message is heard through the word about Christ" – and - Proverbs 4: 23, *"Above all else, guard your heart, for everything you **do** flows from it."* As I have matured in my walk with the Lord, I've come to realize that God never give advice without showing us how to implement His wisdom into our lives.  Philippians 4:8-9 is just one scripture that instructs us on how to guard our heart; as it states, "Finally, brothers and sisters, whatever is true, whatever is noble, whatever is right, whatever is pure, whatever is lovely, whatever is admirable—if anything is excellent or praiseworthy—think about such things. [9] Whatever you have learned or received or heard from me, or seen in me—put it into practice. And the God of peace will be with you." This powerful scripture is the perfect medicine to prevent and eradicate depression. Taking you back to the Old Testament and before the fall of man, mankind's mind &spirit were one with God and man had no evil thoughts. In *Genesis 2:25* it states, "Adam and his wife were both naked, and they felt no shame." Unfortunately, the word of God has been watered down with such legalism in our society today that His word is the last choice we chooses as a solution to walk in divine health or seek Him for the blessings He desire for our lives. In North America we have defaulted to bio-technology, surgery, and medication that allow us to pretend we are walking in great health. Although I have great admiration for the advancements made in the medical industry, I know God has a much better way when it comes to our health. Taking medication to keep your blood pressure normal is not walking in divine health. You see my friend; it's extremely important for you to realize why God want and need you healed and whole. Remember we talked about God gave mankind dominion over the earth and took Himself out of the equation by saying, "Let them have..."? With that command, God still desire things to operate on earth just like things operate in heaven; so let me help you connect the dots. Once you decide to accept Jesus Christ as your personal savior, that simple act gives God the permission to dwell within your body as His spiritual temple. He performs His will on earth through you by supernaturally communicating the instructions to you by your spirit. Pause a minute and ask yourself this rhetorical question, "How can I accomplish God's will for my life being sick or laying up in the hospital? Remember, everything God created has a purpose and all the abilities, talents and gifts are built within the created thing. Here lies your challenge, God is a gentleman and He will never force you to obey Him. Although you may go through periods of not hearing from God, He's always speaking, and meditating on His word will help re-energize your spiritual ears. In spite of His power, God gave mankind a gift called "free will", and He rejoices when we obey Him with a willing heart. As you begin to see God as Abba Father "aka *daddy*", and understand how massively He loves you, your desire to obey Him becomes second nature.

The 2nd statements of truth my coaching sessions are based upon: **The human body is extremely complex, but 100% predictable when it comes to weight loss**. I give the gift of wisdom & knowledge credit for this revelation (I Corinthians 12: 7-10); because it set me free and my desire is to help set you free. Realizing the human body operates like a complex machine with predictability make it very easy to test the body for a particular outcome. This predictability is the main reason we see such advancements in medical practices. Most of my clients and including me before I received this revelation; perceived excessive fat as a problem. Excessive fat is not a problem, it's a symptom. It is a symptom that a few "weight-loss principles" have been broken, and that's the number one task of a healthy lifestyle coach on weight loss; helping clients discover which broken principles are the culprits. Remember earlier we talked about everything in life has principles, and when we apply the principles they produce an expected end. For example, marriages have principles; if you cheat on your spouse, you should not be shocked to find yourself in a divorce court eventually. When it comes to weight loss, I realize it can be a bit deeper than just calories in verses calories out situation, and that's the main reason I wrote this book. Here's the problem you may face like many others; not knowing how your body uniquely respond to nutrients and how those nutrients relates to your daily movement in order to produce the results you desire. Because of this predictability aspect of your body, all weight loss programs should reveal your unique dietary set-point to produce guaranteed weight loss "and" without counting calories. The freedom in such system will unveil the mystery of permanent weight loss tailored for your body. The second major problem is consistently consuming food outside its purpose, and we'll discuss that in more detail in chapter 5.

# Chapter 4: The Purpose of Body Fat

God created body fat with a purpose, just like roaches, mosquitos and flies. For the purpose of this book, we'll leave the insects out of the discussion. God originally created your body to live forever with the ability to heal itself. Unfortunately, you and I lost the right to live forever during the fall of mankind, but your body still has the ability to heal itself to a certain degree given the right nutrients. I personally believe this built-in self-healing power is evidence of God's love and compassion for us. Medical professions understands when disease starts to manifest, your body start making adjustment in attempts to function as close to normal as possible or an attempt to save your life. For example, when you develop an infection, your body temperature increase in attempts to purify or neutralize the infection also known as "a fever" and your white blood cell increase to attack the infection in order to get rid of it. Another example happens when your body goes without food, it enters survival mode by slowing down your metabolism. Although starvation depletes your muscle tissue; the adjustment is designed to preserve energy for your most critical functions: your brain and your heart. When it comes to body fat, your body is not designed to carry it in excess, but body fat has multiple purposes. Body fat helps regulate your reproductive system, body temperature, and assist in keeping your skin, nails & hair healthy as well as store toxin unfiltered by your liver. For the record, these dietary unfiltered toxins have three predominant sources: eating preservative found in foods, consuming genetically modified foods and the effects of chronic stress. Your body will store these toxins in a special type of fat called **"visceral fat"** located in your abdominal region surrounding your vital organs. Although this fat is not visible, the evidence of its presence takes on the appearance of a pregnant woman. This type of fat is not accessible by surgery, and can only be eliminated through a healthy lifestyle change. **Subcutaneous fat** is the second type of fat most people are familiar with. It's the fat you see accumulated on your hips, butt, thighs, abs, arms and back. This fat is typically very pliable and easy to squish between your fingers; unless you are suffering from chronic stress. Chronic stress cause excessive levels of cortisol *(the stress hormone)* in your blood stream and make subcutaneous fat less pliable and difficult to metabolize.

Although you can temporarily eliminate this fat by surgery, a lifestyle change can keep it off permanently.   As you well know, excessive body fat can cause:  heart disease, heart attack, cancer, diabetes, high blood pressure, high cholesterol and other metabolic diseases as well as accelerating the aging process.☹  I am 100% convinced; those are not your fitness goals.

## Chapter 5: Discover the Tri-Fold Purpose

I believe every person on planet earth has a blueprint in their head reflecting what their life "should" look and feel like. If your blueprint does not match your reality, that's a clear indication that something in your life must stop, start or change. Living in the metro area of Georgia, I spend about two hours a day in Auto University. Auto University is using your drive time to listen to motivational speakers or other educational material to help achieve your goals. I recall my coaching mentors *(Tony Robbins)* relate the following concept to depression. He said, "If a person's mental blueprint does not match their reality, AND they are 100% convinced they don't have the resource, talent or ability to make it match, that's when their depression can result in suicide or they become a danger to society." It's no mystery that everybody wants to feel significant and feel certain they are capable of making a difference in the lives of others. As a healthy lifestyle coach, I realize it's extremely important for you to walk in ultimate health to achieve that need. One thing I know for sure; in order to manifest your blueprint into your reality, your "Why" must be bigger than the challenges you will face in the process. That brings me to what I call the "Tri-Fold Purpose" which includes; 1. "Discovering your life purpose", 2. "Discovering your purpose for making the decision to live a healthy lifestyle" and 3. "Discovering the real purpose of food". Getting a handle on these three areas of purpose in my own life sustained me when everything in my life was fighting against my goals and my desire to change.

## **Discovering Your Life Purpose **

Remember the quote from Myles Munroe where he said; "Time is a commodity, and what you do with your time becomes your life!" How many times have someone asked you, "what did you spend your time doing this weekend?" We use time to buy life; that's why it's very important to discover the purpose of your life. Discovering your life purpose will dictate how you spend your time, what you let out of your mouth, what you watch, what you listen to, who you hang out with, how you dress, and most of all how you treat your body. Some people talents and gifts are so pronounced and obvious that it doesn't take a rocket scientist to figure out what gifts they should use towards fulfilling their given purpose. Sadly, many of those people will misuse their gifts and talents if they never discover the true purpose for their life by the Creator. If you're like me, I had to discover my purpose and the journey was quite colorful. Just a quick short story about me: I remember when I was about 10 or 11 years old sitting at the dinner table with my mother and having a casual conversation. It wasn't dinner time or anything of that nature. I clearly remember telling her this; "Mom, I don't know where this is coming from, but I'm going to be responsible for transforming or changing the lives of a lot of people. Although I don't know how I'm going to do it; all I know it's' going to require a lot of my time and have access to a lot of money to do it. I also know I will live in Washington DC or Atlanta, GA; and once I graduate from college I'm not coming back home to live!" She looked me square in the face and said, "I know Lee Lee!" Lee Lee was my childhood nickname and that's another story. At the time of this conversation, I hadn't discovered all the gifts God had given me to vision how this would be possible through my life. After I officially made Jesus the Lord of my life, the Holy Spirit started slowly revealing my destiny to me as I grew in my spiritual understanding. I marvel at how God used the good and bad experiences of my life to manifest His purpose through my life. I honestly believe if He revealed it to me before I was ready, I would have managed to screw it all up. I must say; what a journey it has been, and thank God for His love to correct me along the way.

Our life purpose is designed to solve a problem on earth. Remember in chapter one, we talked about how God use our body to perform His will on earth and that we were born with the gifts & talent required to get the job done? In case you haven't realized it yet, that blueprint in your head about your life was placed there by God. I now realize why so many people are stressed, because they haven't taken the time to discover their purpose. If you fall into this category, chances are you are working a job that you hate, or feel a void you can't seem to satisfy within your life, and it is stressing you out to no end. Please note, your income level is not truly the driving factor, because there have been plenty of millionaires committing suicide. I'm not bringing this to your attention to make you feel bad because most people are in this situation; maybe not to the point of suicide, but miserable enough to affect their health. When I wrote this book, I could count on one hand the number of my friends that believe they are walking in their purpose and making a living doing it. I'm sure as I journey through life I will meet more people walking in their purpose, but most people today are working a job only because the pay is decent or the health benefits are great. Your intentions may have to commit only a year or so, but at some point you became complacent and the next thing you know 10, 15 or 20 years have passed and you're still working the same job and have grown more miserable. Being on this job, it's possible that you are experiencing self-imposed mental stress because deep inside you know this is not where you supposed to be and probably not what you supposed to be doing. In addition to all that, you may not be in the right city, state or region of the country. You may be in a situation where the pay is not quite enough so you've taken on a second job as a solution, but only add more stress. To add fuel to the fire, dealing with toxic superiors, co-workers and rules and regulations being forced on you make life even more difficult. When stress builds up in your body it release a hormone called cortisol. Cortisol is not designed to exist chronically within your human body. It is designed to flood your body in one quick burst in the midst of a life threatening situation giving you fleeing power and then subside. For this reason, helping my clients discover their purpose is a major part of lifestyle coaching because knowing your purpose and operating in it help minimize stress.

I pray this book encourage you to seriously dig deep and discover your purpose. As I have this conversation with clients, a few quickly say things like: raising my kids or "helping people" is my life purpose. Ok that's great, but what happens when the children are grown, they've left the house and you're still living? That season of your life is now over; so what's next? Everybody can use their life to help other people, but it's important for you to know exactly "how" you are capable of helping others. In today's society people are hurting in all kinds of ways, and for many it requires supernatural help to get them delivered from the bondage they've been suffering from over the past few years. Take a minute and ask yourself, "Have I truly discovered my purpose?" Here's a clue: if you hate what you're doing with every cell in your body, you're not operating in your purpose. Here's a "How-To" list to help get you started in the right direction:

1. **Get rid of negative noise in your life to buy back time, and negative noise can be people, places or things**. What I mean by this: watching TV four to five hours a day, hanging out with friend regularly and accomplishing nothing positive for your future, going to bed late but accomplishing nothing and then getting up late, becoming addicted to social media, iPad and smart phone used to play games or watch videos of animals and people doing crazy things. It may be entertaining but not educational or productive for future growth. When you're working two or three jobs trying to make ends meet; who has time to discover purpose? If you never spend quite time long enough to hear the creator speaking to you; discovering your purpose will be a constant challenge.

2. **Meditate on God's promises and His will for your life found in the bible**. How will you know His promises if you never pickup His book to know what they are?

3. **Reflect upon your childhood dreams**. I refer to that as the "pre-fear stage" because I believe they are connected to your purpose in some fashion.

4. **List your "natural" talents**, for example: managerial skills, poetic abilities, musician skills, singing skills, and don't forget life experiences you've overcome. That's a big one to list first, the negative life experiences you've overcome, and the "how" you did it is your gift back to the world. These are the questions I challenge you to ask yourself: What is that "thing" you can do so easily that makes people marvel with such wonder when you're operating in that particular task? What talent or natural ability has been a common thread throughout your entire life? Ladies and gentlemen these natural gifts, and abilities were not given to you for you; they were given to you to be used as an instrument to make the life of someone else better. As it turns out, if you use your gifts, talents and abilities to solve problems for people; guess what, they will be willing to pay you for it….hmmm imagine that! Your gift will make room

for you in the world. I highly encourage you to examine the gifts you've allowed to go dominant. Those are the ones you really need to examine closely because the enemy *(Satan/the devil/Lucifer)* has possibly convinced you to give up on making anything happen with that particular gift. It's a lie so don't believe him, and write it down. As you go through this process, don't just grab a piece of paper and write them down, you need to include the problems your gifts, & talents have the ability to solve for other AND the ordered steps you need to take in making this talent/gift become your profession. After writing the steps down, take action the very next day. Don't let the sun go down each day without you doing something towards the steps you listed. I mean it; make it a TOP priority. It should be first on your daily to-do list as your big rock, and you can thank me later. I'm sure many of you grumbling, murmuring and complaining saying, "I don't know how to do anything else but what I'm doing today", or "I don't have any talents". STOP listening to the devil, he is a deceiver, and the sad part is he typically uses people in your life to whisper these lies in your ear or fool you into believing those thoughts are coming from you; but they are straight from the bowels of hell. You can do all things through Christ who strengthens you. (Philippians 4:13)

5. **List your most dominate life changing passion(s)**. What are you most passionate about that could help someone overcome their struggle in that area. It could be injustice you see happening in your community, and you have resources or skills to help change their outcome.

Now that you have a map on how to discover your life purpose, it's time to exam where you are now. Look at your current life and make a definitive assessment of whether you're on target or not. If you are on target, congratulations! If you are not on target, it's time to take out a piece of paper and devise a plan to get you there. This plan must definitively illustrate the outcome and construct the small steps required to achieve it with definitive time lines, new actions you'll need to take, resources you'll need to take possession of, skills you'll need to perfect, equipment you'll need to purchase or borrow, get the help & support from your love ones by calling a meeting, and most of all; connect with a mentor, someone that's already successful in the area of your desires and goals. Take that mentorship knowledge and tweak it to make it authentically your own. On a side note, if you're working for a company and you've discovered you will need to leave eventually, I wouldn't share this information with them at this time. The best thing you can do for yourself while still working for the company is to obtain the skills, information, or resources you can use as you transition into your purpose. What I mean by that is, while working at this company you may discover a company you never knew exist, a resourceful person, an unfamiliar or a special type of equipment, or prefect new skills you could use to become successful at a faster rate as you walk into your destiny. In the meantime, I advise you to work with a massive load of appreciation and produce excellent work until it's time to turn in your two-week resignation; and you can thank me later! ☺

## **Discovering Your Purpose for Choosing to Live a Healthy Lifestyle**

This is your million dollar discovery process because it's very important to know "why" you've decided to live a healthy life. To be totally honest with you, in today's society it's easier and more convenient to live an unhealthy life. In order for you to make this a permanent transition, your reason must trump all challenges you will face and you must adapt a relentless attitude. For those of you in the fat loss stage, your why MUST be bigger than your plateau, your why MUST be bigger than life sucker punches that will come your way, your why MUST be bigger than any and all types of disappointments. Trust me on this because I'm speaking out of my own experience. Connecting my why to my life purpose compelled me to stop yo-yo dieting. Can you imagine God giving me this mandate and I never figured out how to lose weight permanently? Or how to stay focused in the midst of a major life storm, and let alone when you see me I look like I never visit a gym? I don't think I'd be a very good role model in inspiring others to overcome their weight loss challenges. I realize your "purpose" may not require you to achieve a professional

27

athletic level of fitness, but you still want to be in ultimate health to help other people according to your maximum potential.

Unfortunately, if your reason for making this decision is based on an event, your weight loss will be temporary. Having this discussion with prior clients, I've discovered these few categories that repeatedly result in permanently lifestyle changes: 1. to save their life from disease or sickness, 2. to see the future of their grandchildren live out their lives or 3. to accomplish their purpose for living.

As you ponder over your reason, don't be surprise if you're not ready to make the commitment. In 2006 I had a massive life set-back and it was one of the lowest points in my life. I walked around 3 years looking like the Pillsbury doughboy's wife before I decided to make a physical change towards the end of 2009. Although I knew in my heart I wouldn't stay in that condition; I just delayed making the decision to change. You'll know when you're ready to turn the corner because you will feel it with every cell in your body. In your mind, there will be no other choice and you'll see it as a MUST change NOW mentality, and trust me on this one! If you discover your reason is not sustainable, I encourage you to meditate on this matter to get a clear understanding of the quality of your future if you don't make changes now.

## **Discovering the Real Purpose of Food**

Remember in chapter one, we talked about how God created everything with a purpose? God created food for us with two purposes: first to provide our bodies with *nutrients* and secondly to provide us with *energy*. Your body is designed for movement and a healthy body has the ability to move in various ways. We are not designed to live a sedentary lifestyle, but thanks to the advancement in technology a sedentary life has become much too common. What's important to understand is the purpose of food is still operating regardless of your reason for consuming it. Food does have a language, and we will talk about that in chapters 6 through 8 when we dig a little deeper into the three macro-nutrients: carbohydrates *(sugar)*, protein and fat. Here's the truth, food will never tell you how much it love you, miss you or need you, as it does not have the ability to satisfy an emotional or spiritual deficit. It does however; change

28

your physiology *(breathing & energy level)* to change your state, but you can get the same effect by exercising; just so you'll know!

You see my friend, everything in life operates on a "seed-principle"; meaning you can only reap a harvest based on the seed sown, and the ground in which the seed was sown must be capable of yielding its fruit. A wise farmer never plants a seed without first examining the quality of the seed and the quality of the ground. That means if you need more love in your life, you'll need to sow love into the life of a living being capable of giving love back to you. The most important part of that statement is: "...capable of giving love back to you." I feel very compelled to help you understand that statement on a deeper level. You can apply this concept to relationships, physical or material needs. If a person doesn't possess what you're seeking, they have no way of delivering it to you, because you can't give what you don't have. If love is not dwelling within a person; *for whatever reason*, or a person does not possess the "thing" you need, they can't deliver what you're seeking. You will experience major frustration if you continue to make attempts to reap a harvest from this source. Most people habitually seek to satisfy emotional deficits by drinking alcohol, smoking, or eating carbohydrates as a method of relief from emotional needs or to help calm them down after a stressful event.

Unfortunately these vices are not capable of satisfying those needs, and will result in poor health and massive weight gain. It's no mystery that many people are addicted to carbohydrate *(aka "carbo-holics")* because of chronic stress, and emotional & spiritual challenges. I refer to this as "food abuse" because food is being used outside its purpose. The goal of this book is to help you transform the way you think about food and start using it as a tool to force your body to look, feel and operate according your fitness goals. As you progress through this book, it will help you create vivid pictures in your mind concerning what happens to food once it enters your body and how it relates to your fitness goals. Keeping these images in your mind will help you change your behavior when you're in the midst of food and compel you to make better choices. Remember, the human body is very complex, but 100% predictable when it comes to weight loss.

## Chapter 6: The function of Macro-Nutrient Fat

Dietary fat is broken down into fatty acids once you consume it. Although, dietary fat is an extremely important macro-nutrient to keep in your diet, once I started lifestyle coaching; I discovered many people view fat as "evil". Before we dive into dietary fat, I want to share a report the American Heart Association published generated by the National Institute of Health. This report showed that from 1962 until 2006, obesity in adults age 20-74 more than doubled, increasing from 13.4 percent to 35.1 percent." This rise in obesity has been correlated to the rise in metabolic diseases such as: *diabetes, strokes, heart attacks, high blood pressure, and high cholesterol by the medical professions.* The food industry has made attempts to elevate the problem by manufacturing & marketing "Low-Fat" to "No-Fat" foods. As Americans believed this to be a solution to help overcome obesity, many people adapted the idea that fat is evil. In reality, a few elements of education were omitted in the equation, and the baby was thrown out with the bath water. Just like everything else in life, there are good fats and bad fats. It's very important you know the difference between the two in order to help you make better choices. Initially there were two dietary fat categories; Unsaturated Fat *(good fats)* and Saturated Fat *(bad fats)*, but with the introduction of a process called hydrogenation created another "bad fat" called Trans Fat *(aka Trans Fatty Acid)*. To keep this simple, hydrogenation convert liquid oils *(typically from vegetables)* into a solid, and is designed to increase the shelf life and stabilize the flavor of oils in foods that contain it. If you see the word "hydrogenated" on food labels, you'll know this process was involved and its best to make a different choice. Saturated Fats *(bad fats)* are usually solid at room temperature and derived from animals. To keep this clear in your mind, imagine this is the fat that will "saturate" body fat on your hips, thighs, butt, abs, arms, and back. Just for the record, *I'm not advising you to take meat out of your diet, but it's a good practice to choose leaner cuts and grass fed when possible.*

**Unsaturated fats** *(good fats)* are usually liquid at room temperature and are derived from some fish and vegetables oils such as: olives, avocados, rapeseed, sunflower seeds, other seeds, and nuts. There are two categories of unsaturated fats: monounsaturated or polyunsaturated.   These fats are excellent at raising HDL *(good cholesterol)* and lowering LDL *(bad cholesterols)*.

Here's a list of benefits contributed by consuming unsaturated fat:

- It helps delay hunger sensation forcing you to eat LESS.
- It's required to absorb the fat soluble vitamins *(A, D, E & K)* to move through your blood stream.
- It's required as a pre-cursor to other complex chemical reaction within your body.
- It improves brain function as electrical pulses transmit signals throughout your body's nervous system.
- Improves the biometric integrity of the phase angle.  The "phase angle" is referred to the perimeter of every cell in your body.  Under a microscope, it has the shape of miniature dumbbells arranged closely together; which allow water into your cell to provide nutrients to your mitochondria. Consuming "bad fats" changes the shape of your phase angle and prevents nutrients and water from entering your cells efficiently; as a result, you will experience bloating, loss of energy, and foggy thinking just to name a few symptoms.

Although it's important to have unsaturated fats in your diet, it's extremely important to discovery "your" daily dietary-set point to prevent weight gain due to over eating it.  By the way, coconut oil uniquely consists of medium-chain triglycerides *(MCT)*; which are molecularly smaller and can be used as a backup source of energy in the absence of carbs, and capable of crossing the blood-brain barrier to improve brain function.  The two predominant sources of MCT are human breast milk and coconut oil.

You can now receive your deliverance from thinking fat is "evil".  You only need to remember to consume unsaturated fats *(good fats)* according to your dietary fat-loss set-point.

## Chapter 7: The Function of Macro-Nutrient Carbohydrates

Carbohydrate is the first energy source your body uses for energy by breaking it down into glucose. For complex carbs like; bread, rice, pasta, corn and some vegetables, this process starts immediately in your mouth's saliva by an enzymes called amylase and also found in your pancreas. Simple carbs like, refined sugar and pure sugar requires very little enzymatic reaction for absorption. As carbohydrates travel through your digestive system, additional digestive acids help convert carbs into glucose in preparation to enter your cells. Out of the three macro-nutrients, carbohydrate can be very addictive for many people. Unlike cocaine or other addictive mind altering drugs, you can't live without carbohydrates. If you are addicted to carbs, the solution is to transform your relationship with carbohydrates and consume it based on its purpose, and address the driving force behind the addiction. As your daily dietary set-point for carbohydrate intake is discovered, over eating carbohydrate is eliminated during the course of your 5 to 6 daily meals. As we discussed in chapter five in the section entitled "Discovering the Real Purpose of Food", carbohydrates are not designed to whisper I love you or to satisfy a spiritual or emotional deficits, but it will support & sustain your energy levels on a running program.

## Chapter 8: The Function of Macro-Nutrient Protein

Protein is broken down into amino acids once you consumed it, and is responsible for nearly every task in the life of your cells including its shape, inner organization, and other products manufactured by it like hormones and enzymes. Protein is responsible for receiving signals from outside your cells and mobilizes intracellular responses. It's important for you to understand just how significant protein is to have in your diets; therefore, it's important to keep the explanation simple. Protein is the macro-nutrient responsible for maintaining your muscle mass and rebuilding your muscle tissue. The most popular source of protein is meat based protein. Other protein sources becoming just as popular are plant based proteins as people are transitioning to a more plant based diet to minimize saturated fat. When your muscle pre-maturely runs out of protein from your diet, it starts to metabolize your muscle tissue causing muscle atrophy. Muscle Atrophy is the process of muscle cells depletion causing muscle shrinkage, loss of strength, slower metabolism which results in rapid fat gain. Because your muscle is an active tissue; it burns calories just to exist; therefore, it's important to consume enough protein to accommodate this process. Although everybody needs protein in their diet, the amount required varies from person to person. Men naturally have more muscle mass than woman; therefore, men typically require more protein intake. In addition to gender, a few other factors that dictate daily protein requirement include: your metabolic genetics, your existing muscle mass, the frequency of your movement & intensity, the type of movement such as *strength training vs. cardio,* and medication that can block protein absorption. Once you discovery your daily dietary set-point for protein, over eating protein is eliminated. In chapter 9, we'll talk in more depth about the "vicious cookie cycle" causing a false hunger. Protein has the power to stop false hunger because protein is a very dense in nutrients. It takes your digestive system much longer to breakdown protein; therefore, it delays hunger sensations. As a result, you consume fewer calories. Also protein barely spikes your blood sugar; therefore, sugar cravings are tremendously diminished and fewer calories are consumed. Introducing the right amount of protein in your diet increases the possibility of major fat loss.

## Chapter 9: Factors Preventing Your Weight Loss

Discovering the factors preventing my weight loss set me free when I was on my weight loss journey. During plateaus, I had to evaluate my plan to reveal what factors were causing my failure. As we discuss these factors, take the time to evaluate your current weight loss plan to reveal which of these factor(s) is/are plaguing your weight loss goals. I realize the simple formula of calories consumed vs. calories burned can be a factor, but I want to go a little deeper because the simple solution to that factor is to decrease the amount you're consuming or start an exercise program. If you feel this is the sole reason for your plateau, doing both will help you overcome your challenge much faster. ☺

### **Glycogen Spillage **

What is Glycogen Spillage? Glycogen spillage is created when glucose is in your blood stream **and** all the glycogen stores in your muscles and liver are full; causing glucose spillage to your fat cells. Remember in chapter 7 "The Function of Macro-Nutrient Carbohydrates" where we talked about the digestive pathway of carbs. Let me help you connect the dots and set you free as I paint this picture in your mind. When carbohydrates are consumed, they are converted into glucose. Glucose molecules are small enough to travel in your blood stream and capable of entering the cell walls throughout your body. Every time you eat carbohydrates, your pancreas releases a hormone called insulin into your blood stream to give glucose a ride to your cells. Think of insulin as a taxi cab used to carry the gas *(glucose)* with the destination of putting that gas in the engine of your cells called the mitochondria. The mitochondria is where glucose is used for energy to keep you in motion. The cells in your muscle and liver have little storage tanks called glycogen storage where the mitochondria can access the gas *(glucose)* to keep you energized. Here lies the problem, once all your glycogen storages are full in your muscle & liver, and you continue to eat carbohydrates; your body has no other choice but to store the extra glucose in your fat cells; this process is called "Glycogen Spillage". Remember, body fat is the secondary choice your body will use for fuel; therefore, as you continue to eat carbohydrates your body never get the opportunity

34

to use your fat storage for fuel.  As this cycle continues, weight loss is halted or will continue to accumulate until you stop eating too many carbohydrates or foods easily converted to glucose and start moving. This is why it is extremely important for you to know your carbohydrate dietary set-point to prevent this from occurring.  In case you've wonder why some people can eat carbs all day and never gain a pound, it's because they have a naturally high metabolism.  These individual's metabolism is so fast that as soon as the mitochondria receive the glucose, it use that "gas" pretty quickly, and glycogen spillage never occurs.

While we're on this subject, I want to talk a little on diabetes.  Type-1 diabetics are usually born with it caused by the immune system attacking the pancreas cells responsible for producing insulin. Although the immune system is the root cause for Type-1 diabetics, physicians rarely address the immune system, but are trained to target the symptoms by prescribing insulin.  Type-1 diabetics typically have other immune related illnesses like:  allergies, bronchitis, asthma, and eczema.  On the other hand, if you have type-2 diabetes or know someone with it, I highly encourage you to get a copy of this book to them as a gift of life.  As I've educated myself on type-2 diabetes, I've come to know not all type-2 diabetic victims are overweight, and I wondered, "How can this be possible?"  I have come to understand the elements involved are separate entities.  In the scenario above we talked about a person with a naturally high metabolism capable of eating a large volume of carbs without gaining body fat.  Here's how they can develop diabetes:  each time they consume carbs, their pancreas release insulin and eventually their cells are no longer sensitive to the presence of insulin *(their cells don't hear the "knock-knock" to let the glucose in) or the pancreas start producing less insulin.*  In either case and as a result, glucose is left in the blood stream at high levels and they are now officially a type-2 diabetic.  Although this process is a bit more complex, I want to keep this simple so it resonates with you and encourage you to permanently change your habits.  Do note; these high metabolism individuals will eventually gain body fat if this lifestyle continues because their body is not getting the gas *(glucose)* into the cell's engine *(mitochondria)* for energy.  This same process occurs with overweight type-2 diabetics, especially if they are addicted to carbohydrates causing the "vicious cookie cycle". The vicious cookie cycle is a term coined by Metagenics; it is the inducing of a false hunger due to the rapid drop in blood sugar as insulin is introduced into the blood stream after eating carbohydrates. Real hunger is produced when the brain runs out of essential nutrients *from a nutrient dense meal,* and triggers genuine hunger sensations. Individual addicted to carbohydrate typically have carbs for breakfast; which trigger hunger quicker and more frequent throughout the day as oppose to a person having a protein/fiber based breakfast. "Carbo-holics" usually eat more calories and the sad end to that story is a lack of energy, resulting in no exercise and led to depression due to continuous fat gain. That cycle will continues until the reason for the carbohydrate addiction is broken. If this is your personal challenge, be aware of hidden sugars manufactures are including in foods labeled, "No Added Sugars". A list of hidden sugar names has been included in the workbook to help you identify them in the ingredients. In addition, a food label guide is included in the workbook to help you understand how to read food labels. I encourage you to use these tools to help you make better choices while shopping. One thing you can always rely on; let your taste buds tell you the truth when it comes to foods labeled "No Added Sugar". If it tastes sweet, there's sugar in it, PERIOD! Duly note, as soon as your tongue sense "sweet", your brain kick into action, blood sugar spikes, and insulin is released and you now know the rest of that story.

## **Chronic Stress**

In chapter 5 we discussed how chronic stress prevent fat metabolism because it release cortisol; the stress hormone. To recap that discussion; the chronic presence of cortisol causes a great amount of belly fat called visceral fat. Visceral fat is located in your midsection and very toxic as it surrounds vital organs and give the appearance of a pregnant woman. When these toxins are released into your blood stream, they are carried to the cells of your organs. The cells of your organ are constantly regenerating using the blood it receives; therefore, the function of your organ eventually deteriorate or start to malfunction due to the toxins laced blood received continuously. The general term for these types of condition is called "metabolic disease" and refers to: diabetes, heart disease, cancer, high blood pressure, and high cholesterol. These conditions typically lead to strokes, heart attacks, limbs being removed and eventually death. The only way to get rid of visceral fat permanently is through a lifestyle change by incorporating a balanced diet, exercise and a stress management program. Visceral fat can't be removed by bariatric surgery or liposuction.

## **Loss of Muscle Tissue **

Sarcopenia is a condition referred to loss of muscle tissue, typically due to the aging process. The same process occurs in individuals performing high intensity workouts without an adequate diet to support muscle depletion during the intense workouts. This process also occurs with meal skippers and individual labeled as anorexic. With the exception of the meal skippers, these individuals appear skinny, but when body composition tests are perform, they can have 30% or higher body fat; which is considered obese. I realize that may sound strange to you if you didn't know about this condition, but its' a real problem and it does exist. The group I'd like to focus on for the purpose of this book is the "meal skippers". When I have a "meal-skipping" client, they never understand why they're overweight and can't seem to lose it. These individuals are practicing a miniature version of the sumo-diet. Sumo wrestlers gain massive weight by eating one to two meals a day averaging around 20,000 calories a day. One weight loss principle is to eat 5 to 6 small meals every 2.5 to 3 hours to keep the metabolism high. With each of these small meals, it's important to include the proper serving of protein to maintain muscle tissue. If you are a meal skipper, muscle loss is possible causing your metabolism to slow down which also cause your fat metabolism to slow down as well. This process is also happening if you are consuming too little calories during these 5 to 6 small daily meals. Remember in the "Glycogen Spillage" section above, we talked about glycogen stores are located in your muscle and liver cells? Here's another dot connecting moment; when your muscle tissue is being depleted due to skipping meals or not eating enough protein calories, that means you will have less glycogen stores available. As a results, your body can only tolerate very little carb intake before all glycogen stores are full causing glycogen spillage to your fat cells at a much faster rate. The companion workbook "Operation: Life Re-Map for Divine Health includes a 7-Day Diet Diary. After completing your 7-Day Diet Diary, make an assessment to determine if you are: a meal skipper, protein deprived or eat like a bird.

**\*\*Hormonal Imbalances \*\***

Hormones play a major role in the efforts of burning fat. In addition to controlling other hormones throughout your body, your thyroid is responsible for regulating the rate in which your fat is metabolized. Hypothyroidism is a condition where your thyroid has slowed or stopped functioning properly causing major fat gain. Coupling hypothyroidism with elevated levels of cortisol *(stress hormone)* is a perfect hormonal environment conducive to massive fat gain. If you're suffering from chronic stress, depression may be the reason. If being depressed is true for you; pay attention to how you use food to accommodate depression. It's very common that depression decrease the desire to work out, but the desire for comfort food increase. I encourage you to visualize putting on your workout cloths and head to the gym or park and just start walking, and cast down any images of cake, ice cream and cookies. If you commit yourself to this technique every time you feel stress; working out will become your default instead of grabbing something sweet.

If you are an apple shaped individual, it's possible you suffer from hypothyroidism and/or adrenal fatigue (cortisol) resulting in body fat distributed evenly throughout your body. If you are a pear shaped individual, it's possible you suffer from a sluggish estrogen metabolism and/or adrenal fatigue (cortisol) due to chronic stress. These little team of hormonal imbalances; hypothyroidism, *estrogen & cortisol dominant* prevent efficient fat metabolism in a powerful way. I inherited the "pear shape" and at the age of 50 I discovered I was estrogen dominant while dealing with several stressful situations in my life. In spite of those odds against me, I didn't let my hormonal imbalance stop me from competing in a figure competition in 2016.

My determination compelled me to discover the secret to unlock the mystery of getting rid of my saddle bags and totally reshaped my glutes. That determination and research gave birth to my "30 Day Gut and Butt Fat Blasting System". What I discovered is "the right exercises" mixed with "the right diet" have the power to create a hormonal environment to neutralize this demonic team of hormonal imbalances and force your body to strategically target your saddle bags, thighs, butt and belly fat.

If a hormonal imbalance is involved with your weight loss challenge, here are a few things you can do today to help reverse the effects on fat metabolism:

1. The 30 Day Gut & Butt Fat Blasting System is designed to target stubborn body fat for individual with chronic stress, hypothyroidism, apple & pear shaped individuals, and is accessible at www.bodytransformationsbytrina.com

2. Decrease carbohydrate intake to decrease the release of insulin in your blood stream

3. Implement relaxation techniques or activities like joining a stress management *program* to minimize stress to decrease the release of cortisol.

4. Eat a diet conducive to addressing estrogen dominance like food high in vitamin A or foods that are precursor to the production of vitamin A like: Red or orange vegetables and fruits that are rich sources of beta-carotene.

5. To address thyroid dysfunctions, you have three choices:
   a. Call upon the Kingdom of God for a brand new thyroid through prayer by faith.
   b. Address it holistically by consuming a diet designed to balance the thyroid rich in :
      i. Selenium & Omega 3's like: Fish, Brazil, macadamia & hazel nuts
      ii. A monitored dose of Iodine like: seaweed, iodine supplements
      iii. Vitamin D3 supplementation
   c. Help from your physician

If you a banana shape physique you may or may not have a hormonal imbalance, and just blessed with a naturally high metabolism; *and yes I'm jealous.* On the other hand, it is possible you suffer from another thyroid condition called Hyperthyroidism. With this condition you may appear very thin and have a high metabolism. Although that may sound great to others; this condition can compromise your muscle mass or promote muscle loss if your diet is not sufficient to prevent it. Your challenge may include muscle gain by eating more calories or eat more frequently to maintain existing muscles and build new muscle tissue simultaneously. Unfortunately, you may suffer from sleep deprivation, anxiety, hand tremors, rapid heartbeats and excessive sweating.

### ** Lack of Exercise **

As we grow older, exercise becomes a challenge for many people, but it does not have to be an excuse for weight gain. Remember, the human body operates like a machine and it's predictable. If you can't work out for medical reason and still want to lose body fat, the solution is to discover your dietary set-point to trigger weight loss without an active exercise program. Discovering your dietary set-point for pure fat loss without exercise can be accomplished without compromising your muscle tissue. Although this option is effective, the progress is much slower and eventually you will hit a plateau.

If your reason for not exercising is based on your dislike of exercise, remember; regular exercise will increase the possibility of you independently taking a bath, washing your hair, feeding yourself, getting dressed, using the restroom, getting up without assistance as you continue to age; which will also preserve your dignity. When we talk about lack of exercise, I'm referring to living a sedentary lifestyle. For example; if you are an individual working behind a desk for 8 hours and you never perform deliberate workouts, you are considered to have a sedentary lifestyle.

Here's the truth and I realized this once I became a personal trainer; working out is a blessing. Your body is designed for movement and exercise is a method to keep you operating at optimum levels on a daily basis regardless of your age. By the way, if medical issues are the reason for your lack of exercise; I have good news made possible by Jesus Christ. You can use your faith to get a new hip from heaven. As a matter of fact, you can use your faith to get anything you need from heaven through what I call the "FAITH Bank" (**F**ull **A**ccess **I**n **T**he **H**eaven **Bank**). For non-believers in the faith of Christ, you too can get unlimited withdrawal slips from heaven by accepting Jesus Christ as your personal savior in your heart by faith. Just because you have yet made Him your father, He still loves you as His creation and desires you to walk in divine health.

## ** Medications **

Certain medications interfere with fat metabolism, and this can be very frustrating by putting you in a "Catch-22" situation. I encourage you to check the documented side effects of your medication to help you make the best decision for you and your family. One source I discovered providing such information is www.DrugWatch.com sponsored by the Peterson Firm, LLP located in Washington, D.C. Although medication has prolonged the lives of many people, God's desire is for you to walk in divine health. I am excited and very proud of you for making the decision to live a healthy life and become medication free. If you are a recipient of an organ transplant and your doctor prescribe medication for the rest of your life, God has the power to supernaturally replace organ transplant with a brand new organ from heaven by faith. As you get a clear understanding of God as the great "I AM", you can believe for your healing by faith through the shed blood of Jesus Christ.

## ** Lack of Sufficient Water Consumption **

Water is extremely essential to life simply because an adult body is approximately 65% water; whereas infants are approximately 75% water, as noted by USGS Water Science School. They also concluded that water provide the following benefits for our bodies:

| | |
|---|---|
| <ul><li>Forms Saliva (digestion)</li><li>Keeps mucosal membranes moist</li><li>Allows body's cells to grow, reproduce and survive</li><li>Flushes body waste, mainly in urine</li><li>Needed by the brain to manufacture hormones & neurotransmitters</li></ul> | <ul><li>Lubricates joints</li><li>Regulates body temperature (sweating & respiration)</li><li>Acts as a shock absorber for brain & spinal cord</li><li>Converts food to components needed for survival – digestion</li><li>Helps deliver oxygen all over the body</li></ul> |

No other liquids can take the place of water in fulfilling those responsibilities. When it comes to weight loss, water gives your liver the ability to convert metabolized fat into a water soluble substance to be secreted by your kidneys and excreted through your urine. I have learned a great number of people don't enjoy drinking water. If you fall into this category, I hope this information encourage you to give a new meaning to water and compel you to drink up. Water requirement differs from person to person so here's the basic daily water intake formula: drink half your body weight in ounces per day. For example, if you weigh 120 pounds, 60 ounces of water as a minimum is required per day. Because this formula does not take exercise into consideration, it's important to increase the daily consumption when you work out. Realizing this formula requires a larger person to drink more water on a daily basis can be intimidating. As you incorporate the following trick to overcome this "intimidated" feeling, it becomes easier. This trick reminds me of the old cliché' "How to eat an elephant?; One bite at a time. So here's the trick; immediately upon waking and after using the bathroom, drink a full bottle of the water all at once.

This process will make your body thirsty enough for the rest of the day; making it easier to drink all your water.  The goal of this trick is to force thirst for the rest of the day immediately upon waking.   Using a 200 pound person in this scenario need 100 ounces of water per day. To successfully consume your minimum water requirement will require having your water with you at all times.  If this person water container is 24 ounces; according to the water formula they will need to consume about 4 ¼ bottles of water to meet their daily requirement.

## Chapter 10:  Evaluating the Fruits of Your Spirit

In chapter one, we discovered that everything you can touch, see and feel were created in the spirit before it manifest into the natural realm. This truth is not only responsible for how you feel and the reflection you see in the mirror, but it also holds true for all experiences in every area of your life:  your work life, your daily habits, how you manage your time, & money, and most of all your marriage & family life.  If you're experiencing joy peace and happiness in these areas; then you're on the right track.  If you're experiencing pain, stress and sadness in any of these areas, it's time to discover the root cause. Un-forgiveness is the number one root cause of many health issues as a result of offenses within relationships.   I encourage you to be totally honest with yourself during this evaluation.  Go into this process with the mind set of getting to the root of the problem and stop dealing with the leaves; otherwise, your problem(s) will never go away.  It's very important to make a self-evaluation before examining external factors to determine your contribution to your problem(s).  As you discover your truth, change is inevitable and it will require you to start something, stop something or change something; so brace yourself and be ready.  Here is where I would encourage you to adapt a Kingdom mind-set when re-evaluating every area of your life.  When you think of a king and his kingdom, here's a picture of his environment; nothing is ever out of place and that includes his home, vehicle, office, kitchen, and garage.  A king dresses with dignity; not just his cloths, but his mind-set as well.  His children are reared with proper manners; he surrounds himself with gifted people in areas where he is not; he is respected by his community, and he is never broke because he owns everything.  The following five topics with guidelines will help you progress through your evaluation process:

### * Evaluating Your Current Career Choice *

How to determine if you've chosen the right profession?  If what you are doing for a living allows you the ability to use your natural gifts and talents, you may have made the right professional choice, and the opposite is also true.  Chances are if you are in the right profession, I imagine your job doesn't really feel like a job; you look forward to each day, and you probably would do it free if you are in a financial position to do so. Some of you may be doing it free of charge right now by participating in an outreach ministry with your church. On the other hand, those of you operating in the "wrong" professional choice are probably experiencing the opposite, but there is hope. I can clearly remember when I was working for a major insurance company in Atlanta, Ga. I knew I wasn't where I was supposed to be and I most definitely was not doing what I was born to do. My stress levels were through the roof, and I would physically make myself sick on Sunday nights at just the thought of having to walk into that building Monday morning. As I grew in my relationship with Christ, that feeling of being in the wrong profession became stronger and stronger until I left the company in July 2004. After making this leap of faith, I suffered a few rough times and I could have return because I did leave the company in good standing, but I couldn't go back in my heart. As it turns out, that was the best decision I could have made because it allowed me to give birth to God's purpose for my life.

If you haven't by now, this is a good time to grab a piece of paper and devise a plan to get you where you want to be. I know that sounds simple and easy, and believe me that is the easy and simple part. The difficult part is the day-by-day steps and dedication it requires to get you there. The one thing I do know is that it can be done IF YOU BELIEVE you can do it. Why is this so important in weight loss? The answer is simple...it will be a major stress eliminator for you. Your outlook on your current job will change. You will begin to see your job as provision to your vision or a means of perfecting a skill you'll need when operating 100% in your purpose. All of a sudden, your co-workers will see you coming to work with a skip in your step and a smile on your face. Why, because you know it's just a matter of time, you will be operating 100% in the purpose you were born to fulfill. You will be the head and not the tail; you will be the lender and never borrow (Deuteronomy 28:12-13).

## * Evaluating Your Daily Habits & Rituals *

Now that you've discovered you're in the wrong profession, what do you do now? Earlier I touched on the power of habits, and I gave a clear understanding that habits have an expected end. Once you know where you want to be, your daily habits should be arranged in such a way that leads to the results you desire. Re-evaluating your daily rituals & habits are not only required to get you in the right career, but also required to activate the healthy lifestyle principles revealed in chapter 11. Refer to the factors preventing weight loss as discussed in chapter 9 to help reveal your habits contributing to your weight loss failure. For example: If you eat carbohydrate based foods (rice, pasta, bread, dessert, potato chips, cookies, donuts) every day and skip any aerobic activity, you can expect to have excessive body fat. To reach your fitness goals or make a change in your career, some of you may need to call a family meeting to inform or warn them about the changes that is about to take place within your life. This may also involve cleaning out your kitchen cabinets, refrigerator and freezer to reflect a winning environment. You may need to connect with a mentor or enroll in a class for a career change. By the way, if you decide to revamp your kitchen cabinets & freezer; please donate the foods to your local food pantry. I realize the food you donate may not be healthy, but starvation trumps weight loss issues.

I learned something very powerful from one of the seminars of my coaching mentor; Tony Robins. He said if you don't know how to do something, find someone that has already achieved success in the area you want to achieve success, and follow their blueprint. It's important to tweak a few elements to fit your personality, but follow the principles. In other words, don't try to reinvent the wheel because success has a road map. Establishing the right habits you already know that will work, gives you a sense of certainty that you will meet your goal and help decrease any anxiety you may have in accomplishing those goals. In the field of weight loss, your daily habits should look a little like this: drinking "pure" water in ounces based on half your body weight, eating a balanced diet reflecting your movements & genetics, exercising with a combination of aerobics and resistance training frequently and consistently, and keeping a positive outlook on life. If you have other social habits that have contributed to your failing health or weight gain like: smoking, drinking alcohol in excess, getting only 4 to 5 hours of sleep daily, not working out at all, food addictions, hanging out with toxic friends and walking in un-forgiveness, those things MUST stop, and NOPE they are not up for negotiation; PERIOD!

### *How You Spend Your Time*

As I've conducted many weight loss consultations, not having enough time to meal prep or exercise is the top reason clients believe contributed to their inability to lose weight. What's ironic about this excuse is the consultation typically reveals major time wasting activities they've committed to. I want to share with you a line of questions to ask yourself: What's your favorite TV shows? What time do you get up and what time do you go to bed? How far do you have to drive to get to work? What time do you have to be at work? What time do you typically get home from work? Do you work on the weekends? How often do you get to talk to your friends? What method of communication do you use when talking to your friends and family? Do you cook your meals or do you go out for meals? How often do you go out to eat? These questions will immediately reveal that not having enough time is a major deception. I realize when you have a family to take care of; you will not have as much "free-time" as a single person. Learning how to delegate duties and re-mapping your priorities will help you tremendously. Time wasting activities are time wasting activities regardless of being single or married. For example, spending hours gossiping with a friend or family member, staying up until 11pm to 12am watching TV are a waste of time; especially watching the bad news tube. Staying up on current events is important, but constantly watching and listening to demonic acts committed within the world starts building fear within your spirit, and alters your outlook on your life. Here are a few suggestions to help you re-map how you spend your time: Google the event in particular to by-pass all the fear based stories that can put you in a negative state; tape your favorite shows and play them on the weekends while you prep your meals. I challenge you to a TV-fast to reveal just how much you can achieve during the fast. I took the TV-fast challenge in 2009 and have been TV free ever since; it was the best thing I could have done for myself.  Not only was I able to spend more time to improve and mature my walk with the Lord, but time to sharpen my skills and talents to give back to the world on a whole new level.

Sleep deprivation is another activity that can wreak havoc on time and your ability to lose weight.  During consultation I usually hear things like; "I just can't go to bed early; I have so much to get done before I go to bed; or I only need a few hours to sleep".  Here's the reality if you've decided to thrive on 4 to five hours of sleep; sleep deprivation wreak major toil on your body in stealth mode.  Sleep is important for all your physical systems.  This is the time your body restores and repairs itself, but if you never give your body time to complete the restoration process; inflammation remains, cortisol levels will rises, blood pressure elevates, brain fog increase, and sadly lack of energy increase.  Remember when you were a child, your parents had you in the bed early with the lights off and you went to sleep?  As an adult, you can re-condition your body back to that state by simply making the decision to stop reading in bed, turn off all lights & illuminated devices, stop social media activities, remove the pets from your bedroom and turn off the TV.  If you have a TV in your bedroom, moving it to another room can help eliminate temptations.  Here's my advice, establish a designated bedtime and stick to it regardless of any un-done chores.  Prioritizing your daily life (personal & business) can save your life, your sanity and lead to better health due to less anxiety and stress.  In order to re-map your life for more time, it's important to understand "how" to manage your time according to your goals.  This is very critical when making a career change, improving your health, improving your marriage, family relationship and any other areas of your life.  Here are few suggestions:

**1. Call a meeting with your loved ones and *let them know the changes you are about to embark upon; share the details and explain how this decision will impact your relationship.*** You may discover a friendship overhaul will be required.  These are friends & family members that make you feel emotionally and spiritually drained when you're in their presence or communicate with them.  I'm not suggesting to get rid of them; only you can make that decision.  These are individuals that don't qualify to be in the front row of your life's theater. Making this decision alone will help you lose weight because it will help eliminate stress. You'll be amazed at how freeing you will feel by making this simple change, and knowing you have a life filled with optimistic, positive & spirit filled friends in your inner circle. I realize this suggestion can be a little scary and challenging for you, but just be faithful to your new commitment. I also want you to be prepared for the doubters in the beginning, but don't let that shake you. Stay focused, be positive and relentless because as they see your level of commitment & massive progress; they'll want to join your party.

**2. Designate a "Me-Time" and stick to it.** This is the time you designate to exercise, prepare your meals, study for your new degree or certification, attend a class, meet with a mentor or soak in your relaxation program. This is the one area I find most people; especially women, fail to make this a priority when transcending to live a healthy lifestyle. I understand why many people place "me-time" last on their priority list; because it appears to be a selfish act. In reality, not making this a priority is the ultimate selfish act, because when you fail to take care of you or choose not to become more skillful, or more resourceful; not only will you not be available to help others, but you will not be able to give back at your highest potential. The key to this step is to be consistent & relentless; when life throws you a curve ball, deal with it; keep moving; and never stop. I pray you adapt a life mission to die empty!

**3. Set a definitive deadline to accomplish each phase of your new re-map plan.** For example; how many pounds you'd like to lose by a certain date, a dress size or pant size you'd like to fit in or the date in which you want to graduate and receive that new degree. The key to this step is to make it measureable, achievable and realistic while taking into consideration your current household responsibilities.

**4. Create a daily-to-do list.** This list should include something towards your new goals in addition to your normal responsibilities. Make sure your big rock activities are first on the list, and you are your big rock. The key to this step is to eliminate stagnation of growth; avoid distractions, stay in gratefulness, focus on your goals and most of all operate in love. This is a guaranteed way to see progress, and progress fuels motivation and builds momentum.

**5. Organize your closet, food pantry, refrigerator, office space, garage and any other area of your life that's in disarray.** The whole purpose of this step is to re-arrange your external environment to match your new purpose filled organized inner you. Remember your external is a reflection of your internal state of being. By committing to this step, one immediate advantage is saving money; you'll know when you've truly ran out of an item to prevent buying unnecessarily, and you'll stop losing items in your home or office. Making this a lifelong commitment will allow you to keep your eyes on peace and build your desire to live methodically. As you grow and become more connected with your spirit; this concept will become clearer.

**6. Celebrate your accomplishments.** Set up a reward system for each completed phase; make certain the reward or celebration event is aligned with your ultimate goal. This will refuel you, give you something to look forward to along your journey and keep you in the game; and the next thing you know "BAM", you've achieved your goal.

### *How You Manage Your Money*

When it comes to weight loss, many clients believe income is a contributing factor to their inability to lose weight. In my experience working with these clients, it doesn't matter if they work in a warehouse on 3$^{rd}$ shift barely making minimum wage or a business owner driving a Porsche. A few of my low income clients believe it cost too much to live a healthy life. In reality, it cost much more to become unhealthy especially with the cost of medication and surgeries.

On the flip side of the financial coin, my high income clients feel they don't have time to run their business; meet job responsibilities and worry about what they eat and finding time to work out. Although this group eat out often because it's more convenient; the truth is restaurants provide healthy choices; committing to choose them is the challenge.

Money most definitely has an impact on your ability to invest in quality whole foods. I recall being in that same dilemma not too long ago; short on money and no health insurance. My heart bleeds for single parents because I'm sure it's a hundred times more challenging when you have other mouths to feed.  Re-mapping how you manage your money could help you discover money to apply to better quality foods, weight loss coach, personal trainer, or other life goals.  I want to share these suggestions for limited income as well as having an abundant income:

### *Limited Income:*
So how can you overcome the money challenges when you're on a shoe string budget and still desire to live a healthy lifestyle?  Grab your workbook and write your re-map money management mission statement.  I encourage you to be 100% honest with yourself as you progress through this process.  Every person blows some level of money, and that level is relative to the amount of consistent income coming in versus the carnal desires money is used to satisfy.   I'm just as guilty; the only difference now is I have a "Play Money" category in my budget giving me 100% control on how much I spend on play activities.  Life is too short to eliminate fun from your life.  The important rule about fun is; it must lead to more life, joy, peace, and love for you and others you share your life with.

To help solve your money management challenge; it's important to know how and where you're spending your dollars.  Investing in financial software like Intuit Quicken is a great tool I used to reveal my truth.  I'm not affiliated with this company in any way; therefore, my suggesting it is not putting any money in my pocket.  I know this software has the ability to allow you to create any spending category of your desire.   If you know of different software that can accomplish the same goal; by all means use it or invest in it.  Take your workbook and refer to the habits you noted in question 15 to help you devise your list.  This list should refer to the habits that require money to sustain; especially those that have contributed to any sickness, weight gain, marital problems, and failing business such as:  cigarettes, alcohol, excessive dining out, emotional clothes shopping, illegal drugs, porno, magazine subscriptions, useless club memberships, and website memberships I think you get the idea.  For those with children, I encourage you to add unnecessary toy purchases, or other unnecessary indulges they really can do without.

Notice, I haven't mention junk food because I want to expound upon that a little deeper. You see junk food purchase is a sneaky little rascal that has a way of making you forget you even indulged in its evil seductions. You know what I'm talking about, those impulsive stops at fast food joints for a small order of fries, or quickly grabbing a snicker bar at the checkout counter, swinging by Star Bucks for that special latte with caramel and whipped cream, the number of trips to the vending machine during work hours. I realize this may seem nick picking, but trust me; the numbers don't lie. You will be utterly surprise at how fast they add up; I know I was shocked when I committed myself to this challenge.

The next step is to take your list and create categories in the software according to your purchases. This step is a little tedious and will take some time to get comfortable with, but it is worth your time. This step will also require you to hold on to your receipts; especially cash transactions, until you can log your transactions into the software. In addition, you must decide when the best time to enter the data: as it happens; at the end of your day; weekly, etc. Vending machine purchases will require you to remember to add them daily; otherwise, you will forget you made that purchase. After consistently doing this for one month, you can create a pie chart report reflecting the percentage of income being used in each category. Trust me; you will be shocked as it was a jaw dropping moment for me when I did this back in 2000. Now that you have a visual of where you've been spending money you can see where you can make the shift. For some, the percentage of spending will show pretty significant and for others maybe not so much. The whole goal of this task is to encourage you to stop unnecessary spending in order to make money available to invest in a healthy lifestyle and items you need to make your career adjustments. How wonderful it would be knowing you have the money to enroll in a class conducive to your career adjustments; purchase more fresh or fresh frozen foods; join a gym (actually go to the gym); invest in a personal trainer (and obey his/her commands), and or invest in a fat loss program designed to teach you how to feed your body for the rest of your life. Taking these steps will build hope in your spirit like never before, and you can see yourself winning.

In addition to building hope, taking this step will also eliminate mindless spending. That's the power of financial & dietary journaling; over time you will eventually stop making unnecessary purchases and stop investing in things not conducive to your fitness goals. Here's the biggest nugget to take into consideration when it comes to money management; if you have identified your purpose for living, and your ultimate fitness goals; let those desire dictate how and where you spend your money.

### *Abundant Income:*
Having an abundance of income brings on a different weight loss challenge, and the solution is a simple shift in your priorities. Although having an abundance of income allow for more options, it's still important to manage your money; therefore I recommend taking the steps previously mentioned to expose how and where you're spending your money. As you review your spending and the priorities within your business & life, I want to expose the many options available to you through your abundance:

- Invest in a weight loss coach for permanent weight loss.
- Hire a personal chef to cook and prepare your meals is just a simple phone call away.
- Hire a personal trainer; the sky is the limit for you!
- Outsource work responsibilities to free up time for workout or to learn a new skill.
- Invest in a business mentor for hands on experience

Here's the question I challenge you to ask yourself: How can I efficiently use my income to buy back time in order to improve my health and/or transition into my life's purpose? As you conduct your evaluation, remember these wisdom keys: a chef is not a weight loss coach; therefore, learning how to feed your body for permanently weight loss requires the expertise of a weight loss coach. To accelerate your weight loss progress, investing in the right personal trainer is just another phone call away.

Having such abundance gives you the power to surround yourself with people that will dance by the beat of your "new" life re-map healthy lifestyle drum. You are "The Shot-Caller & Big-Baller", and you can be that in every area of your life.

**\*Evaluating the Dynamics of Your Marital/Family Atmosphere\***
Single readers please do not skip this section. Sit back, relax and take in a deep breath as I help you understand why. Many of the issues discussed in this section are real issues married couple experience, and being single does not exempt you from experiencing the same. Being single simply means you don't have a spouse, but you do have individuals in your life that can force these same challenges upon you. For that reason, I encourage you to listen; besides I'm sure you have the desire to be married at some point in time just as I have. As I published this book in 2017, I was 51 and never been married. It wasn't because I had no desire to be married, or never fallen in love. You see I asked God to intervene supernaturally in my relationships to guarantee I make covenant with the right man capable of going where He (God) sends me. I transferred this authorization to Him because I understood just how important it is to choose the right spouse. I've come to realize it's important to date someone long enough to discover their character when you're in the middle of a storm and witness how they respond. If you decide to make the same decision and transfer this authority to God; be 100% sure that's your desire because He will follow through. I made the mistake of disobeying His voice and all I can say, "I pray to never make that mistake again; ever!" Thank God for His mercy and forgiveness because God is for us & not against us. His thoughts are higher than our thoughts. He knows the future; therefore, you and I can put our trust in Him. When it comes to choosing a spouse; God leaves that totally up to you. He may orchestrate the two ships passing in the night scenario and dangle them in your presence, but He will never make the choice for you. The way you transfer relationship authority to God is to follow His written word, and receiving knowledge & wisdom from the Holy Spirit as He guides you. In this process, I recommend asking God to activate the gift of discernment when it comes to your marriage candidate.

With all that being said, marriage is the one area of your life that has the power to wreak havoc on your health. That havoc doesn't solely come from a place of domestic violence, infidelity or financial incompatibility.  It can simply be a difference in lifestyle or body typing, and for the purpose of this book; we will focus on that area of contribution.

Before we dive into lifestyle & body type incompatibilities; I do want to acknowledge the effects of domestic violence, infidelity and financial issues.  When you look at the dynamics of marriage, it welcomes the one person on the planet you've grown to trust outside your maternal family.  You have given this person 100% access to your most intimate thoughts and space.  Once that trust has been betrayed in the form of infidelity, and domestic violence; many negative events can and usually take place:  divorce, suicide, murder, alcoholism, becoming a shopaholic, workaholic, drug use and other vices that destroy marriages, health and life itself.  Surviving this type of situation has the power to rip ones soul and forgiveness is key.  Forgiveness will set you free, and I encourage you to leap into forgiveness as quick as possible; because if you choose not to forgive, God can't forgive you either.  God made this very clear to us in Matthew 6:15 as it reads, "But if you do not forgive others their sins, your Father will not forgive your sins.

In spite of all the craziness in the world, I'm happy to say there are marriages that are strong and keeping things moving. Weight loss challenges is an area where getting the right blue print tailored for the family is the key, and it starts with conducting a family meeting.  My experience counseling married couples revealed these most challenging weight loss factors:  difference in metabolism, jealousy & insecurity, individuals that love obesity, and incompatible lifestyles.


### Differences in Metabolism:
One of the most difficult scenarios is when your spouse has an extremely high metabolism and can eat any and everything on the planet and NEVER gain a pound.  Taking them out back and beating them like a Persian rug is not the stance you want to take.  It's important to show them love, because they are not out to sabotage your weight loss efforts.  As you learn how to relate to them in this area, you'll discover they really want to support you and see you achieve your fitness goals. This is the time where massive

communication is extremely important and must be done in a peaceful atmosphere. Losing weight can be very emotional; especially for woman. Once you decide to have the "talk", it's important to leave out ALL accusation phrases like: 'You Make Me...', 'every time I...' or 'every time you', accompanied with the pointed finger, hand on the hip and the snake like head movement. If you take that stance, be ready for major resistance and zero support because that creates an offensive atmosphere, when you're really looking for compassion. You must communicate with a compassion seeking mentality when you decide to have the conversation and say phrases like: "how you feel when...", or "will you help...". Your plan may include agreeing to remove any foods from your freezer & cabinets that do not promote a healthy lifestyle. This solution is very important if you've discovered you are an emotional eater. As you transcend into a healthy lifestyle, keeping your kitchen filled with healthy food choices is the key to permanent change. Life is too short to never indulge in your favorite treat. Once you've reached your fitness goals, you and your significant other can periodically schedule a date night and indulge in your favorite treat together. Who knows, that could lead to a little calorie burning romance later☺.

### *Jealousy & Insecurity:*
The second scenario I see in couples centers around jealousy and/or insecurity from the other person. In this situation, it doesn't seem to matter if the other person needs to lose weight too, but the jealous/insecure person has a high tendency of sabotaging the weight loss process in fear of losing them to someone else. The best solution is to assure them of your love in a manner that resonate with them. You know your spouse; therefore, only you can determine what method will influence them the most. It's important to compassionately walk them through your future, if you continue on an unhealthy path. Remember, behind every principles lies a promise. I want to walk you through a scenario that supports this fact. Let's say you've been diagnosed as a type-2 diabetic; which is a lifestyle induced condition and 100% reversible. Without a lifestyle intervention, type-2 diabetes can result in: blindness, amputation of your arms, legs, fingers & toes. Having diabetes does not prohibit the

function of your menstrual cycle or your digestive system; therefore, you're still capable of having a monthly period, bowel movements, urinating and releasing gas. If your diabetes eventually results in blindness or amputation of any limbs; the questions you need them to answer are: How will they get you to the restroom and will they assist in the clean up? You can expect the room to become very silent, but wait for the answer. If the dynamics of such conversations does not change their mind-set concerning your future, I encourage you to develop a petition prayer requesting God to give them a new heart straight from heaven and bind the spirit of fear.

### *The Love of Obesity:*
I realize this may come as a shock, but there are some cultures and a few people I've encountered that are attracted to obese individuals; in their eyes the bigger the better. From the individuals I've encountered with this mentality, that attraction usually stems from their childhood where they received tremendous attention, love and affection from someone with an obese physical characteristic. As a result, they developed a behavior of attraction to someone of that statue. The solution for this scenario requires deep spiritual reprograming through petition prayer, and the suggested prayer topics include binding the spirit of: rejection, abandonment, loneliness, fear, and a revelation that love has no size or color. In addition to prayer, having the same conversation mentioned earlier would be appropriate in this scenario. I realize the solutions presented appear simple in nature, and I also realize it is not; but I do know it's possible through faith in God.

### *Incompatible Lifestyles:*
Incompatible lifestyle among couples is a clear example that opposites do attracts. One enjoy eating any and everything under the sun; whereas, the other desire to make more healthy choices. When you factor in the need to lose weight; you must develop a plan to keep you permanently on track. First, call a meeting and involve them in your decisions. The challenge you'll need to overcome involves deciding who will:
- Shop for groceries and what items to purchase.

- Cook the meals and will separate meals be prepared

Living a healthy lifestyle requires more kitchen time for food prep and cooking, so take that into consideration if you decide to prepare two separate meals each day.  Restaurant choices can be a solution or a challenge depending upon how you approach it.  If you both agree to pick a restaurant that provide the options to make healthy choices as well as unhealthy choice, you can still win.  The challenge is actually making the choice to choose the healthy entrées.


### *Exercise:*

Exercise is another area where couples can be incompatible.  When it comes to exercising, some couples tend to be hot or cold on the matter; either they love it or hate it.  All too common, many couples tend to work out less as they grow older or rarely work out together for various reasons.  If exercise is not a part of your life, I encourage you to assess why.  Unless you're paralyzed from the neck down, exercising is possible by getting in contact with the right personal trainer to help you through mechanical challenges.  A simple walk in the park will get you going in the right direction, and a great bonding moment. If your spouse has not bought into the exercise idea, don't give up on them.  The key to bring your spouse on board is to consistently share your progress with them.  Nagging is not the technique resulting in influence; nagging results in resentment, hostility, impatience, and a guarantee you'll continue to work out alone.  By simply sharing your progress; I 'm certain they'll eventually want to join you because they wouldn't want you to start looking younger and being able to out run them in a race.  Once they come aboard, you can help them establish their own fitness goals like: increase their strength, speed, agility or flexibility.  The principle of encouragement fuels one to push harder, stay the course and get massive results.

### *Incompatible sleep pattern*:

Incompatible sleep pattern among couples is another area to overcome. Living a healthy lifestyle involves getting at least 7 to 8 hours of sleep daily, but many couples have a difficult time turning everything off and simply going to bed. Some of the reasons I've heard during consultations are: "my life is a little more complicated than most people"; "I have deadlines to meet"; "I have kids"; "I just don't have enough time to get everything done during the day! The solution to this problem involves you making a definitive decision to simply go to bed. Making rest a priority and remapping your daily activities will maximize your time as you become more productive within a 24 hour period. Refer back to the section entitled, "How You Spend Your Time", and implement those time management solutions.

To add fuel to this fire, **snoring** is another sleep robber for couples. The solutions to this problem may require you to partner with a sleep professional. Although there are many over the counter devices that can help; they only address the symptom of snoring. My advice is to go to a professional to discover the root cause of snoring and address the cause. I am no professional, but I do understand and know sleep apnea is a medical condition where snoring is a symptom. As a health coach, and knowing what I know about sleep apnea, you want to address that immediately. To reverse sleep apnea requires a lifestyle change. If you or someone you know have been diagnosed with sleep apnea, please make note that the C-Pap does not get rid of **or** reverse sleep apnea. It's simply a device used to keep a constant flow of oxygen to the brain when the patient stops breathing frequently throughout the night.

These last two areas of lifestyle incompatibility among couples can be very complex and require a major shift in the mind-set; **drinking alcohol and smoking.** If you and your spouse are plagued by these as an addiction; encouraging each other to quit will be a challenge. For this reason, I encourage you to seek intervention from an addiction specialist. For the purpose of this book, I want to focus on drinking and smoking as an occasional activity. When it comes to weight loss:

- Alcohol is filled with empty calories; meaning high calories, but no nutritional value causing weight gain.

- Alcohol also creates an acidic state within your body, and all diseases thrive in an acidic state.
- Alcohol also prevents the body from metabolizing fat efficiently.

These are things to take into consideration if you use alcohol as a means to relax after a hard day of work. If you're in the "fat loss" stage of your fitness journey, I encourage you to eliminate alcohol at 100% until you've reached your goal. If you decide against 100% elimination of alcohol, you can still reach your goal, but the progress will be much slower, discouraging and disappointing.

Smoking on the other hand does not interfere with fat metabolism directly, but it does hinder cardio vascular advancement while exercising for weight loss. I know you would agree that breathing is important. Remember in chapter 10 in the section entitled "Evaluating Your Daily Habits & Rituals" we revealed that every habit has an expected end; well it definitely applies to smoking. In addition to cancer and death, smoking:
- Accelerates the aging process
- Causes an offensive odor to some people
- Creates a sense of isolation at work, in restaurant and sometime bands your presence all together
- Increases insurance rates in some cases
- Interferes with your ability to date certain people

As you commit to living a healthy lifestyle, I will agree with you in prayer to lose your desire to drink and smoke.

## Chapter 11: Starting Your Healthy Lifestyle Journey

As you've progressed through the course of this book, you should have discovered the root cause of your weight loss challenges. The best way to overcome these challenges is better education and discovering solutions that are unique to your weight loss challenge. As a healthy lifestyle coach, I present this book to educate you and direct you to the right solutions tailored for you. My desire is to allow this book give you hope, clarity and an infallible map to win your weight loss battle.

Now that you've uncovered the root of your weight loss challenge, it's time to devise a plan. Remember, the first step is to call a family meeting and announce this permanent shift you are about to embark upon to explain how it will affect them. If you have weight loss sabotaging friends in your life, I encourage you to first make a mental shift concerning your relationship, and be prepared to re-arrangement them in your "life's theater" according to their reaction. If you discovered that working too many hours has been a major contribution to your weight loss goals, I suggest speaking with your boss to let him/her know you've decided to save your life, and share the changes that will involve your job. It's important to let the boss know the quality of your work will not decline in the process, but will improve as your health improves.

### **Preparation is the Key**

Here's where the rubber meets the road through the vice of preparation. To live a healthy lifestyle preparation is the key and the old cliche' "If you fail to plan, then you plan to fail" is 100% applicable during this journey. Here's the truth, preparation is a must regardless of the complexities of your life. I realize the more responsibilities you have the more difficult it will be, but you can do all things through Christ who strengthens you. *(Philippians 4:13)*.

The next few sections will cover the elements required for permanent weight loss and activities that lead to a healthy lifestyle. We will cover the 7 basic healthy lifestyle principles that must be active, the three life certainties, understanding how meal prep can make this lifestyle easier, understanding the rules of grocery store shopping and the dynamics of exercise options.

## **Daily Healthy Lifestyle Principles**

Regardless of your life complexities, these seven healthy lifestyle principles MUST be active in your life:

1. Eat within 30 to 40 minutes upon waking. Exception: if you work out 1st thing in the morning, a fasting-work out is best and have your 1st meal *(or protein shake)* after the workout.
2. Eat every 2.5 to 3 hours to consume 5 to 6 **small** meals a day: breakfast, mid-day snack, lunch, afternoon snack, dinner and possibly another small protein/veggie snack 2 hours before bed time.
3. Drink at least half your bodyweight in ounces of water per day; more on workout days.
4. Never skip meals: Eat fresh or fresh frozen foods according to your daily dietary set-point eliminating preservatives, genetically modified foods, fried foods and fast foods.
5. Consume your last meal at least 2 hours before bed time.
6. Exercise 4 to 5 times per week with a mixture of cardio and resistant training according to your fitness goals.
7. Achieve 3 to 4 bowel movements per day. Four elements affecting bowel movement are: consuming 10 to 12 servings of category 1 vegetables, adequate water consumption, exercising regularly and consuming unsaturated fats *(good fats)* according to your daily dietary set-point.

I encourage you to look at your life in reference to these principles and devise a plan to incorporate these principles according to the complexity of your life.

## **Three Life Certainties**

If living a healthy lifestyle seems too impossible, here are three life certainties that will set you free and allow you to prepare with ease. Every human being on the planet will experience the following three certainties throughout the day: Waste Elimination *(solid, liquid or gas)*, Thirst and Hunger. If you do not experience all three of these events more than once a day, you are headed to some form of disease.  So here's how using these certainties can help you in your preparation:

- ***Waste Elimination*** – The only preparation you need for this certainty is to know where the restrooms are or leave the room to pass gas when among strangers, your friend, family or co-workers; unless you're rocking some sick contest…right fellas? *Ladies, in case you didn't know, some guys are notorious for those types of contests, and it's not for us to understand…just know some do!*

- ***Thirst*** – Living a healthy lifestyle requires adequate water consumption and no other liquid takes the place of water. Remember in Chapter 9 we talked about how the lack of water can prevent fat loss?  During that section we discussed the trick used to force thirst for the rest of the day by drinking a full container immediately after using the restroom upon waking up in the mornings.  To successfully consume half your bodyweight in ounces of water per day, you'll need to take it with you.  You can accomplish this in one or two ways: investing in a refillable container or purchase enough disposable containers.  Regardless of your choice, you must have your water container with you at all times.  This is especially important when visiting a facility for the first time, and you're not sure if water will be available.  Once you make your container decision, create a timed bench mark to finish each round.  After doing this consistently over the next 7 to 14 days, your body will automatically trigger thirst sensations, eliminating the need for timed alerts.

- ***Hunger*** – As I write this book, I'm 51 years old and I have never received a phone call or had a conversation with someone that said, "Trina, guess what?  Girl, I got hunger yesterday, can you believe it?"  Unless this person has been sick and a loss of appetite was a part of the illness, I would think this person was drinking alcohol or smoking a funny cigarette.  Getting hungry is not a surprise; therefore, there's no reason to not prepare or plan ahead for this certainty. Once you determine what time you need to leave home, how long you will be away from home and when you return will dictate which meals you'll need to pack.  In order to achieve healthy lifestyle principle number 2 as stated in the previous section *(eating every 2.5 to 3 hours),* taking your meals with you will guarantee success.  The more stable your life, the easier this principle is to incorporate.  For example, if you are a stay at home parent or work out of your home, or work a 9 to 5 job reporting to the same building using the same desk it's easier to designate a place to store your food and establish a designated time to eat.  You'll just need to make sure your co-workers and family members dance by the beat of your new healthy lifestyle drum.  If you've been a meal skipper, chances are they are conditioned to see you skip lunch or not take snack breaks.

If your work life involves frequent traveling within your community as an outside sales person or require extended stay traveling; the more challenging it is to incorporate this principle, but not impossible.  The solution is to overcome the uncertainties of traveling is to establish the right mind-set, develop a fool proof plan and follow the plan relentlessly.  As a healthy lifestyle coach, I've been coined as "The Excuse Buster".  In 2006, I suffered a major set-back in my life and balloon to 167 pound; I'm only 5'1".  By the end of 2009, I was still working as a benefit counselor traveling domestically coast to coast mainly during the fall seasons.  It was during that time I made a decision in my heart to change the image in the mirror.  I was done with avoiding the mirrors in my home, wearing black all the time, hiding from old friends and staying away from the gym because I was embarrassed about my weight.  I became relentless about losing weight and traveling was not an excuse; as result, I lost about 40 pounds in 90 days while traveling.  Once I starting lifestyle coaching, I realized I was offering a few of those tricks and secrets to my traveling clients as solutions.  For that reason, I published another book entitled, "How I lost 40 Pounds in 90 Days While Traveling".  All the tricks and secrets I created & discovered during this process were used to create the blue print I revealed in the book.  If traveling is a contributing factor to your weight loss challenge, then I encourage you to take advantage of the book.  All you have to do is adapt a relentless mind-set and follow the blue print within to achieve your weight loss goal relentlessly.☺

## **Meal Prep**

The solution to hunger is to meal prep according to where you will be when you consume the meal and your fitness goals.  Meal Prep – is cooking/preparing all your meals for an entire week on one designed day of the week, and packing them in such a way making it easy to grab every morning.  I find the best practice is to repack your lunch bag every night before going to bed.  Many fitness athletes I'm acquainted with meal prep on Sundays, and so do I.  The day you choose doesn't matter, you just need to make it happen consistently every week.  As I mentioned earlier, considering where you will be when it's time for your meal dictates what's possible, and secondly the meals must be conductive to your fitness goals.  Here's a list of questions you must ask yourself during meal prep:  Does the meal require refrigeration and will one be available?  Does it require microwaving before consumption, and will one be available?  Is it very portable?  Is the smell offensive in regards to the environment, because popping open a can of mustard covered sardines in a conference meeting is probably not a good idea.  Meal prep is the best way to prepare for hunger.   Not only does meal prepping guarantee your food is available, but it keeps you in control of the ingredients.  Here's what I mean by selecting foods according to your fitness goals:  Let's say you work 8 hours behind a desk, and you've chosen not to work out, but you still want to lose weight.  Snacking on too many foods easily converted into glucose *(bread, corn, rice, pasta, fruits, popcorn, soda, coffee w/sugar, and carrots)* is not conducive to your weight loss goals.  In order to make this decision, you'll need to know your dietary set-point to make weight loss happen, and pack your food according to your dietary set-point.

## **Grocery Store Knowledge**

In chapter 10 – Evaluating the Fruit of your Spirit required evaluating the contents of your refrigerator and kitchen cabinets. I'm sure you discovered a few items to donate to your local food pantry. Living a healthy lifestyle will requires more trips to the grocery store as you will consume more fresh or fresh frozen foods. This is another area to consider when managing your time and discussing the requirements of this change during the family meeting. If you haven't called the family meeting, it's important to conduct one to make sure your efforts are successful. In the event you appoint a family member for these grocery trips, please share these four grocery store healthy lifestyle rules with them:

1. ***Never grocery shop hungry*** – otherwise this will increase the possibility of snacking on samples offered by the store not conducive to your weight loss goal. Trust me on this one, because I'm speaking from experience.

2. ***Never grocery shop without your grocery list*** – if you forget your main item and you already have a tight schedule, getting back to the grocery store will be a major challenge and increases the possibility of getting off track with your preparation goals.

3. ***Shop the perimeter of the store*** - this is where the fresh and fresh frozen foods are located because they require refrigeration. Although this is where most healthy foods are located, a few items like: fruit juice, salad dressings and frozen & dried fruits require a closer examination. Fruit juices located in this area sometime have extra sugar added. The only way to discover added sugar is by examination of the label. The same holds true with salad dressings; manufactures sometimes add hidden sugars and the only way to discover it is by examination of the label. For the life of me, I will never understand why manufactures add sugar to dried fruits and frozen fruits, but it happens and I advise you to check the label. Please make this pledge to yourself if you've purchased milk, fruit juice, canned fruit, salad dressings from the center of the grocery store un-refrigerated, STOP IMMEDIATELY! As a matter of fact, if you have some in your refrigerator or cabinet,

pack it up and give it to your local food pantry.  These items are loaded with preservatives to increase shelf life.  Remember, preservatives are toxins, and toxins prohibit your body from metabolizing fat efficiently, and contributes to visceral fat.

4.  ***Always read food labels*** – there will be times when access to fresh foods is not an option.  Understanding how to read food labels is a must; therefore, refer to the food label guide included with this book.  The first 3 ingredients listed are the most abundant ingredients.  To maintain ultimate health and to lose body fat, it's important to avoid foods listing the following as the first three ingredients:  sugar, salt, saturated fats and any preservatives.  We talked about the "hidden sugars" manufactures add to foods.  Remember, just let your taste buds tell the truth and compare the ingredients to the hidden sugar list included with the book.

## **The Impact of Exercise**

Exercise is your ticket to faster results, and it has so many benefits.  As I've grown older, I realize what a blessing it is to exercise.  In chapter 9 we talked about hormonal imbalances and how the stress hormone cortisol prevents fat metabolism.  The best solution to eradicate cortisol out of your blood stream is to flood it with endorphins.   Endorphins are hormone secreted within your brain & nervous system that are released during high intensity exercise producing a number of physiological effects. As endorphins eradicate cortisol out of your blood stream, it also relieves pain and induces a feeling of pleasure similar to morphine.  Although exercising will not solve the source of your depression, it will get you closer to your fitness goal as a side effect and change your state to feel more "happy".

Here's what I've discovered throughout my fitness journey, you can use exercise and dieting to synergistically force your body to perform and transform exactly as you picture in your mind.   For example, if you want to perform like a professional football player, performing sport specific exercises with the proper diet can help you out perform other player choosing not to take advantage of this knowledge.  Have you ever seen a fat loss transformation picture of someone initially shaped like the Michelin man and the after photo look like a smaller version of the Michelin man?  That individual failed to reshape the body by introducing weight lifting.  In order to reshape a body, building muscle by weight lifting will accomplish that, and you must eat because starvation will not build a muscle.

Exercise has the following benefits:  burn fat more efficiently, keep your bones strong, increase relaxation, you sleep better, give you more energy, improves your skin, improves your mood, reverse the aging process, increase your metabolism, your cloths will fit you better, and these are just a few awesome benefits.  If you haven't been working out, you can decide today.  I encourage you to discover what will help you get off the couch.  There are so many options to choose from such as:  getting a personal trainer, investing a DVD to workout at home, join a fitness club and participate in group class, join a local boot camp class, start a walking group in your neighborhood, start a fit-bit community.  The sky is the limits; you just need to decide...today!

## Chapter 12: The Dieter's Prayer

Towards the end of 2011 I made a definitive decision to compete in my first fitness competition. During that time I wrote "The Dieter's Prayer" modeled after Matthew 6: 9-13 as a pledge to myself, and I wanted to share it with you. I encourage you to create your own pledge or embrace this one as support for your fitness journey. What I love most about this prayer is; it helped me transform my mind-set to live a healthier life, and I pray it does the same for you. As I stated early on, God want and need you healthy to victoriously perform His will through your life. With God, Him, all things are possible; just trust in Him and watch God perform a miracle in your life and health:

*Intimate Praise and Worship* - Our Father which art in heaven, Hollowed be thy name: Our Heavenly Father, you are my creator and the creator of every beast of the fields, and every fowl of the air, and every fish of the sea, and every creeping thing that creeps upon the earth. You are the creator of our body; a vessel designed to be your temple with your Spirit dwelling within us. We come to you with thanksgiving for you are the great God and the great King above all gods. We thank you for every beast of the earth, every fowl of the air, and every green herb grown as meat to nourish our body temple. We thank you for the creation of the universe to set balance on earth as a place for your earthbound kingdom children to dwell and marvel with wonders.

*Praying God's Will* - Thy Kingdom come, Thy will be done in earth, as it is in heaven: Father, we confess that instead of worldly use, we will allow you to use our body as a temple to perform your will on earth just as your will is done in Heaven. We confess to use our authority to keep our bodies in good health by consuming food grown from the earth, and keeping our bodies in motion. We confess to calling upon your name for strength and guidance to live a long life.

*Praying for your Needs* - Give us this day our daily bread: Holy Spirit, help us to transform our mind to understand we are the administrator of this body and not the owner. As the administrator of this body, we require the proper finance to gain access to live, organic foods. We need the wisdom to understand the nutritional labels created by the manufactures. We need a powerful voice to change and eliminate the use of pesticides, insecticides and the creation of genetically modified foods. We need wisdom to influence healthy changes within our family as well as our community and country.

*Forgiveness* - **And forgive us our debts, as we forgive our debtors:** Father, thank you for forgiving our sins, and the repeated patterns resulting in health failures due to: walking in un-forgiveness, maintaining toxic relationships, speaking failure & death in the life of others as well as ourselves; eating dead fried & processed foods, & foods high in fat; carbohydrates addictions, drinking alcohol, smoking cigarettes, taking drugs, lack of exercise, lack of rest for our body & mind, and most of all not feeding our spirit with Your Word daily. Father we forgive those that deceive us with false "healthy" advertisement for the foods we purchase to feed our families. We forgive the medical & pharmaceutical industry for concealing the healing powers of your land as a mean to stay healthy. We forgive those responsible for passing laws and making mandates on how food is manufactured and grown causing a slow death to our bodies. Father we forgive all those that cause an offense to us and our families; known offenses and the unknown offenses.

*Pray for Protection* - **And lead us not into temptation but deliver us from evil:** Father we ask that you order our steps and help us control our tongue. We thank you for our assigned angelic hosts that camps around us 24/7 providing supernatural protection. Father we thank you for favor, discernment of spirit and deliverance from any and all evil actions against us; known and unknown.

*Kingdom Praise & Worship* - **For your Kingdom is the power and the glory, forever Amen:** You are the creator of the earth and you are the King. You are the God & King of Heaven and earth. You will reign forever throughout eternity. We adore you as our One True God & King, in Jesus' name, Amen!"

How to connect with the author, Trina Claiborne:

Sign up for free monthly newsletters at:
www.BodyTransformationsByTrina.com

Book for speaking events:
www.BodyTransformationsByTrina.com/book-trina-now

Free One Hour Consultation:
www.bodytransformationsbytrina.com/consultation

Email:  BodyTransformationsByTrina@gmail.com

Phonel:  706-383-7222

Fax:  678-828-5865